Brain Embryology and Congenital Brain Malformations: Conventional and Advanced Neuroimaging

Editors

THIERRY A.G.M. HUISMAN
AVNER MEODED

NEUROIMAGING CLINICS
OF NORTH AMERICA

www.neuroimaging.theclinics.com

Consulting Editor
SURESH K. MUKHERJI

August 2019 • Volume 29 • Number 3

ELSEVIER

1600 John F. Kennedy Boulevard • Suite 1800 • Philadelphia, Pennsylvania, 19103-2899

http://www.neuroimaging.theclinics.com

NEUROIMAGING CLINICS OF NORTH AMERICA Volume 29, Number 3
August 2019 ISSN 1052-5149, ISBN 13: 978-0-323-68246-6

Editor: John Vassallo (j.vassallo@elsevier.com)
Developmental Editor: Casey Potter

Neuroimaging Clinics of North America (ISSN 1052-5149) is published quarterly by Elsevier Inc., 360 Park Avenue South, New York, NY 10010-1710. Months of issue are February, May, August, and November. Business and editorial offices: 1600 John F. Kennedy Blvd., Suite 1800, Philadelphia, PA 19103-2899. Business and editorial offices: 6277 Sea Harbor Drive, Orlando, FL 32887-4800. Periodicals postage paid at New York, NY, and additional mailing offices. Subscription prices are USD 397 per year for US individuals, USD 653 per year for US institutions, USD 100 per year for US students and residents, USD 451 per year for Canadian individuals, USD 832 per year for Canadian institutions, USD 525 per year for international individuals, USD 832 per year for international institutions and USD 260 per year for Canadian and foreign students and residents. To receive student/resident rate, orders must be accompanied by name of affiliated institution, date of term, and the *signature* of program/residency coordinator on institution letterhead. Orders will be billed at individual rate until proof of status is received. Foreign air speed delivery is included in all *Clinics* subscription prices. All prices are subject to change without notice. POSTMASTER: Send address changes to *Neuroimaging Clinics of North America*, Elsevier Health Sciences Division, Subscription **Customer Service, 3251 Riverport Lane, Maryland Heights, MO 63043. Telephone: 1-800-654-2452 (U.S. and Canada); 314-447-8871 (outside U.S. and Canada). Fax: 314-447-8029. E-mail: journalscustomerservice-usa@elsevier.com (for print support); journalsonlinesupport-usa@elsevier.com (for online support)**.

Reprints. For copies of 100 or more of articles in this publication, please contact the Commercial Reprints Department, Elsevier Inc., 360 Park Avenue South, New York, NY 10010-1710. Tel.: 212-633-3874; Fax: 212-633-3820; E-mail: reprints@elsevier.com.

Neuroimaging Clinics of North America is covered by *Excerpta Medical/EMBASE,* the RSNA Index of Imaging Literature, *MEDLINE/PubMed (Index Medicus),* MEDLINE/MEDLARS, SciSearch, Research Alert, and Neuroscience Citation Index.

PROGRAM OBJECTIVE

The goal of *Neuroimaging Clinics of North America* is to keep practicing radiologists and radiology residents up to date with current clinical practice in radiology by providing timely articles reviewing the state of the art in patient care.

TARGET AUDIENCE

Practicing radiologists, radiology residents, and other healthcare professionals who utilize neuroimaging findings to provide patient care.

LEARNING OBJECTIVES

Upon completion of this activity, participants will be able to:

1. Review the role of diffusion tensor imaging (DTI) in the evaluation of brain connectivity, development, and white matter diseases.
2. Discuss magnetic resonance imaging (MRI) as an imagining technique used in the evaluation of normal brain development in neonates and infants.
3. Recognize the use of fetal MRI in the diagnosis of brain abnormalities and migrational disorders.

ACCREDITATION

The Elsevier Office of Continuing Medical Education (EOCME) is accredited by the Accreditation Council for Continuing Medical Education (ACCME) to provide continuing medical education for physicians.

The EOCME designates this enduring material for a maximum of 9 *AMA PRA Category 1 Credit*(s)™. Physicians should claim only the credit commensurate with the extent of their participation in the activity.

All other healthcare professionals requesting continuing education credit for this enduring material will be issued a certificate of participation.

DISCLOSURE OF CONFLICTS OF INTEREST

The EOCME assesses conflict of interest with its instructors, faculty, planners, and other individuals who are in a position to control the content of CME activities. All relevant conflicts of interest that are identified are thoroughly vetted by EOCME for fair balance, scientific objectivity, and patient care recommendations. EOCME is committed to providing its learners with CME activities that promote improvements or quality in healthcare and not a specific proprietary business or a commercial interest.

The planning committee, staff, authors and editors listed below have identified no financial relationships or relationships to products or devices they or their spouse/life partner have with commercial interest related to the content of this CME activity:

Anthony James Barkovich, MD; Matthew J. Barkovich, MD; Sonia Francesca Calloni, MD; Luca Caschera, MD; Mario A. Cedillo, MD; Jacob P. Deutsch, MD; Mary Fowkes, MD, PhD; Thierry A.G.M. Huisman, MD; Alison Kemp; Beth M. Kline-Fath, MD, FAIUM; Pradeep Kuttysankaran; Avner Meoded, MD; Jena L. Miller, MD; Shashidhara Murthy, MD; Suresh K. Mukherji, MD, MBA, FACR; Thomas P. Naidich, MD; Charles Raybaud, MD, FRCPC; Javin Schefflein, MD; Mariasavina Severino, MD; Fabio Maria Triulzi, MD; John Vassallo.

UNAPPROVED/OFF-LABEL USE DISCLOSURE

The EOCME requires CME faculty to disclose to the participants:

1. When products or procedures being discussed are off-label, unlabelled, experimental, and/or investigational (not US Food and Drug Administration [FDA] approved); and
2. Any limitations on the information presented, such as data that are preliminary or that represent ongoing research, interim analyses, and/or unsupported opinions. Faculty may discuss information about pharmaceutical agents that is outside of FDA-approved labelling. This information is intended solely for CME and is not intended to promote off-label use of these medications. If you have any questions, contact the medical affairs department of the manufacturer for the most recent prescribing information.

TO ENROLL

To enroll in the *Neuroimaging Clinics of North America* Continuing Medical Education program, call customer service at 1-800-654-2452 or sign up online at http://www.theclinics.com/home/cme. The CME program is available to subscribers for an additional annual fee of USD 244.40.

METHOD OF PARTICIPATION

In order to claim credit, participants must complete the following:

1. Complete enrolment as indicated above.
2. Read the activity.
3. Complete the CME Test and Evaluation. Participants must achieve a score of 70% on the test. All CME Tests and Evaluations must be completed online.

CME INQUIRIES/SPECIAL NEEDS

For all CME inquiries or special needs, please contact elsevierCME@elsevier.com.

NEUROIMAGING CLINICS OF NORTH AMERICA

FORTHCOMING ISSUES

November 2019
Spine Intervention
Majid Khan, *Editor*

February 2020
Psychoradiology
Qiyong Gong, *Editor*

May 2020
Magnetoencephalography
Roland Lee and Mingxiong Huang, *Editors*

RECENT ISSUES

May 2019
Headache and Chiari Malformation
Noriko Salamon, *Editor*

February 2018
Temporal bone Imaging: Clinicoradiologic and Surgical Consideration
Gul Moonis and Amy Fan-Yee Juliano, *Editors*

November 2018
Ischemic Stroke
Lotfi Hacein-Bey, *Editor*

SERIES OF RELATED INTEREST

MRI Clinics of North America
Available at: www.Mri.theclinics.com
PET Clinics
Available at: www.pet.theclinics.com
Radiologic Clinics of North America
Available at: www.Radiologic.theclinics.com

THE CLINICS ARE AVAILABLE ONLINE!
Access your subscription at:
www.theclinics.com

Contributors

CONSULTING EDITOR

SURESH K. MUKHERJI, MD, MBA, FACR
Professor, Department of Radiology,
Michigan State University, East Lansing,
Michigan, USA

EDITORS

THIERRY A.G.M. HUISMAN, MD
Professor of Radiology, Neurology,
Neurosurgery, and Pediatrics, Edward B.
Singleton Department of Radiology,
Texas Children's Hospital, Houston, Texas,
USA

AVNER MEODED, MD
Assistant Professor of Radiology, Pediatric
Radiology and Neuroradiology, Johns Hopkins
School of Medicine, Johns Hopkins All
Children's Hospital, St Petersburg, Florida,
USA

AUTHORS

ANTHONY JAMES BARKOVICH, MD
Professor in Residence and Chief of
Pediatric Neuroradiology, Neuroradiology
Section, Department of Radiology and
Biomedical Imaging, University of California,
San Francisco, San Francisco, California,
USA

MATTHEW J. BARKOVICH, MD
Clinical Fellow, Neuroradiology Section,
Department of Radiology and Biomedical
Imaging, University of California, San
Francisco, San Francisco, California,
USA

SONIA FRANCESCA CALLONI, MD
Department of Neuroradiology,
San Raffaele Scientific Institute, Milano,
Italy

LUCA CASCHERA, MD
Postgraduation School in Radiodiagnostic,
University of Milan, Milan, Italy

MARIO A. CEDILLO, MD
Department of Radiology, Icahn School of
Medicine at Mount Sinai, New York, New York,
USA

JACOB P. DEUTSCH, MD
Department of Radiology, Icahn School of
Medicine at Mount Sinai, New York, New York,
USA

MARY FOWKES, MD, PhD
Department of Pathology, Director of
Neuropathology and of the Mortuary Service,
Icahn School of Medicine at Mount Sinai,
New York, New York, USA

THIERRY A.G.M. HUISMAN, MD
Professor of Radiology, Neurology,
Neurosurgery, and Pediatrics, Edward B.
Singleton Department of Radiology, Texas
Children's Hospital, Houston, Texas, USA

BETH M. KLINE-FATH, MD, FAIUM
Professor, Department of Radiology, Cincinnati
Children's Hospital Medical Center, Cincinnati,
Ohio, USA

AVNER MEODED, MD
Assistant Professor of Radiology, Pediatric
Radiology and Neuroradiology, Johns Hopkins
School of Medicine, Johns Hopkins All
Children's Hospital, St Petersburg, Florida,
USA

JENA L. MILLER, MD
Assistant Professor, Department of
Gynecology and Obstetrics, Johns Hopkins
University, Baltimore, Maryland, USA

SHASHIDHARA MURTHY, MD
Department of Radiology, Icahn School of
Medicine at Mount Sinai, New York, New York,
USA

THOMAS P. NAIDICH, MD
Director of Neuroradiology, Professor of
Radiology, Neurosurgery and Pediatrics,
Irving and Dorothy Regenstreif Research,
Professor of Neuroscience (Neuroimaging),
Department of Radiology, Icahn School of
Medicine at Mount Sinai, New York, New York,
USA

CHARLES RAYBAUD, MD, FRCPC
Emeritus Professor of Radiology (Pediatric
Neuroradiology), University of Toronto,
Toronto, Ontario, Canada

JAVIN SCHEFFLEIN, MD
Department of Radiology, Icahn School of
Medicine at Mount Sinai, New York, New York,
USA

MARIASAVINA SEVERINO, MD
Neuroradiology Unit, IRCCS Istituto Giannina
Gaslini, Genoa, Italy

FABIO MARIA TRIULZI, MD
Neuroradiology Unit, Fondazione IRCCS Ca'
Granda Ospedale Maggiore Policlinico, Milan,
Italy

Contents

This article discusses the normal anatomy of the posterior fossa structures followed by a discussion of the characteristic neuroimaging features of a variety of cerebellar and brainstem malformations. In this context, the authors classify posterior fossa malformations based on the neuroimaging pattern into (1) predominantly cerebellar, (2) cerebellar and brainstem, and (3) predominantly brainstem malformations.

The spine and spinal cord are composed of multiple segments initiated by different embryologic mechanisms and advanced under different systems of control. In humans, the upper central nervous system is formed by primary neurulation, the lower by secondary neurulation, and the intervening segment by junctional neurulation. This article focuses on the distal spine and spinal cord to address their embryogenesis and the molecular derangements that lead to some distal spinal malformations.

Disorders of the ventral induction give rise to a group of congenital malformations that share in common the failure of the prosencephalon cleavage and subsequent formation of midline structures, presenting with a wide spectrum of severity. This article focuses on the imaging findings of the holoprosencephaly spectrum and septo-optic dysplasia, their epidemiology, embryology, and the common clinical associated anomalies. Knowledge of the imaging features of these disorders is necessary for a correct interpretation of findings and accurate parental counseling. Diagnostic evaluation of patients should include molecular screening and genetic counseling to characterize prognosis and risk of recurrence.

Diffusion tensor imaging (DTI) is an advanced MR imaging technique that provides noninvasive qualitative and quantitative information about the white matter microarchitecture. By measuring the three-dimensional directional characteristics of water molecule diffusion/mobility, DTI generates unique tissue contrasts that are used to study the axonal organization of the central nervous system. Its applications include quantitative evaluation of the brain connectivity, development, and white matter diseases. This article reviews DTI and fiber tractography findings in several brain malformations and highlights the added value of DTI and fiber tractography compared with conventional MR imaging.

A new neuroimaging dimension is currently being adopted. The structural connectome reveals macroscale white matter connectivity of the human brain, providing insights into brain networks organization. Connectomics (analysis of the connectome) has potential for elucidating aberrant networks (eg, in congenital brain malformations, especially axonal pathfinding disorders). Connectomics provides a powerful set of network measures, which can serve as noninvasive biomarkers for the diagnosis, prognostication, and treatment response of children. We discuss the principles of connectome reconstruction and visualization of the pediatric structural connectome using current state-of-the-art neuroimaging and postprocessing techniques, and we describe potential connectomics applications to study brain malformations.

Corpus Callosum: Molecular Pathways in Mice and Human Dysgeneses

Charles Raybaud

The corpus callosum is the largest of the 3 telencephalic commissures in eutherian (placental) mammals. Although the anterior commissure, and the hippocampal commissure before being pushed dorsally by the expanding frontal lobes, cross through the lamina reuniens (upper part of the lamina terminalis), the callosal fibers need a transient interhemispheric cellular bridge to cross. This review describes the molecular pathways that initiate the specification of the cells comprising this bridge, the specification of the callosal neurons, and the repulsive and attractive guidance molecules that convey the callosal axons toward, across, and away from the midline to connect with their targets.

Foreword

Brain Embryology and the Cause of Congenital Malformations

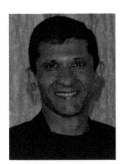

Suresh K. Mukherji, MD, MBA, FACR
Consulting Editor

When I see a patient with a congenital malformation of the brain or spine, my first thought is "Oh My Gosh"! Well...not really, as it would not be appropriate to publish what I am really thinking. Then, my "go-to" person is usually on vacation or at a meeting! So, I was delighted when my friend and colleague, Dr Thierry Huisman, agreed to edit this issue, and I was thrilled when I saw the final product.

Drs Huisman and Meoded have created a wonderful blend of topics that review the normal embryology of the brain and spine and explain how arrests in embryogenesis result in the congenital malformations. This approach will improve our understanding of these difficult subjects and help demystify these complex conditions. They also have articles on more advanced topics, such as connectomics and molecular mechanism for dysgenesis.

This is a superb issue, and I am very grateful for the world-class authors who agreed to contribute to this issue. The articles are beautifully written, and the illustrations are exquisite. Finally, I want to thank Drs Huisman and Meoded for creating such a detailed, up-to-date, and comprehensive issue. This will certainly be a wonderful reference that can be used by both radiologists and clinicians in their daily practice. Quite frankly, I can't wait to start reading it!

Suresh K. Mukherji, MD, MBA, FACR
Department of Radiology
Michigan State University
846 Service Road
East Lansing, MI 48824, USA

E-mail address:
sureshkm@msu.edu

https://doi.org/10.1016/j.nic.2019.05.002
1052-5149/19/© 2019 Published by Elsevier Inc.

neuroimaging.theclinics.com

Preface

Brain Embryology and Congenital Brain Malformations: Conventional and Advanced Neuroimaging

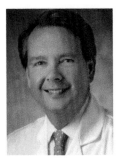
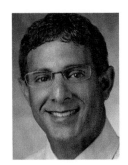

Thierry A.G.M. Huisman, MD   Avner Meoded, MD
Editors

This issue represents an overview of the multimodality neuroimaging approach of the normal and abnormal developing pediatric brain.

The significant and continuous development of different neuroimaging techniques has revolutionized the evaluation and understanding of multiple congenital brain malformations over the last 2 decades. The number and complexity of recognized congenital brain malformations have steadily increased. Multiple "new classifications" have been proposed based on neuroimaging findings. Increasing image resolution and the inclusion of prenatal neuroimaging allow us to refine and achieve the correct diagnosis. Moreover, advanced neuroimaging techniques (eg, diffusion tensor imaging and connectomics) allow us to better study and understand the microstructure and "wiring" of the normally and abnormally developing brain.

For a better and complete understanding of brain malformations, a multidisciplinary approach is mandatory, involving experts from neuroembryology, neurogenetics, neurochemistry, pediatric neurology, and pediatric neuroradiology.

The outstanding contributions in this issue discuss the key role of conventional and advanced neuroimaging techniques in the evaluation of normal brain development and in the diagnosis of congenital brain malformations. We aim to present a detailed, up-to-date, comprehensive body of information that can be used by both radiologists and clinicians for their daily practice and may stimulate scientific interest.

We are thankful to Suresh K. Mukherji, MD, MBA, FACR, Consulting Editor of the *Neuroimaging Clinics*, for inviting us to be guest editors for this special issue.

Last, but not least, as guest editors, we have been very fortunate that multiple world-renowned experts in the field accepted our invitation to share their knowledge and expertise with us. We are sincerely grateful to all the authors for the invaluable excellent contributions. This work would not have been possible without their invaluable help.

Thierry A.G.M. Huisman, MD
Department of Radiology
Texas Children's Hospital
6701 Fannin Street, Suite 470
Houston, TX 77030, USA

Avner Meoded, MD
Department of Radiology
Johns Hopkins All Children's Hospital
501 6th Avenue South
St Petersburg, FL 33701, USA

E-mail addresses:
huisman@texaschildrens.org (T.A.G.M. Huisman)
ameoded1@jhmi.edu (A. Meoded)

neuroimaging.theclinics.com

MR Imaging of Normal Brain Development

Matthew J. Barkovich, MD, Anthony James Barkovich, MD*

KEYWORDS

• Brain development • Pediatric brain • Normal brain • Neurodevelopment • Pediatric neuroradiology

KEY POINTS

- Normal brain development is best assessed by MR imaging.
- Fetal sulcation lags behind premature neonates of equivalent gestational age.
- Myelination generally progresses from central to peripheral, dorsal to ventral with sensory axons myelinating before motor axons.
- MR of the brain has a near adult appearance by 2 years of age.
- Tiny lactate peak on MR spectroscopy is normal in term neonates.

INTRODUCTION

One of the important functions of MR imaging in neonates and infants (and, to a lesser extent in fetuses) is its use to evaluate brain development. Development is measured by many different parameters: (1) in the fetus, important metrics include the sizes of brain structures (ventricular size, cerebral biparietal and cerebellar transverse, and anteroposterior vermian diameters), degree of sulcation, volume of white matter, ventricular morphology and size, and formation of the interhemispheric commissures; (2) in the first 2 postnatal years, assessing normal brain growth and development involves evaluating the rate, location, and extent of myelination, the continued development of the corpus callosum and the cortical sulci and gyri, the proper proportions of the regions of the mid-hindbrain (both by measurements and by relative sizes), and, sometimes, the relative degrees of growth of the different structures of both forebrain and hindbrain structures. Adequate assessment of these features requires a detailed understanding of normal brain development. Although a full discussion of brain development is well beyond the scope of this article, the authors herein describe findings on MR imagings of fetuses (18 weeks and older), neonates, infants, and children up to about age 8 years; even though the brain at this stage is still not completely mature as identified by molecular or quantitative MR imaging analyses, the changes are too subtle to identify by qualitative MR imaging. Quantitative microstructural evaluation of white matter maturation is beyond the scope of this article.

THE FETAL BRAIN

The fetal brain is too small to be imaged using current MR imaging techniques until about 18 weeks gestational age, at which time the structures become sufficiently large to evaluate by MR imaging. The main difference between the fetal brain and the brains of prematurely born babies at equivalent postconceptional age is that sulci develop earlier in babies born prematurely than in fetuses of the same postconceptional age who are born at term.[1] In fetuses, the brain can first be evaluated well at 16 to 18 weeks; however, at this age, the brain and fetus are still quite small and the fetus can be very active, impeding the assessment of many abnormalities.[2] If it is

Disclosure Statement: The authors have nothing to disclose.
Neuroradiology Section, Department of Radiology and Biomedical Imaging, University of California, San Francisco, 505 Parnassus Avenue, Room S257, San Francisco, CA 94143-0628, USA
* Corresponding author.
E-mail address: James.Barkovich@ucsf.edu

Neuroimag Clin N Am 29 (2019) 325–337
https://doi.org/10.1016/j.nic.2019.03.007
1052-5149/19/© 2019 Elsevier Inc. All rights reserved.

necessary to perform scans this early in gestation, multiple acquisitions are often necessary to obtain diagnostic images. As the fetus grows through the second trimester and early third trimester, motion progressively diminishes and, after ~30 weeks, the quality of images is often quite good due to increased fetal size and consequent decreased mobility. Our usual technique involves acquiring single slice fast spin echo images in the sagittal, axial, and coronal planes, supplemented with diffusion imaging and, sometimes, with a cine technique to assess fetal motion. If initial imaging suggests hemorrhage, gradient echo or susceptibility-weighted images (SWI) are also used to confirm the blood and its extent. It is important not to mistake the large areas of germinal matrix still present in younger fetuses near the ventricular ependyma for blood; blood will "bloom" on SWI but germinal matrix does not.

At 16 to 18 gestational weeks, the images may be grainy due to the small brain size. The cerebral cortex is still quite smooth and the layer of underlying white matter quite thin (Fig. 1). Relative to the cerebral mantle, the ventricles are relatively large at this age, but measurements show that they remain about the same size throughout gestation, becoming relatively smaller (and therefore appearing smaller) as the cerebral mantle enlarges. The corpus callosum seems short, the germinal matrix is still fairly thick and hypointense relative to the cerebral mantle, basal ganglia and thalami are poorly seen, and the cerebellum is not much larger than the brain stem (which has a fairly mature appearance).

By 18 to 20 weeks, significant expansion of the cerebral white matter can be detected, with relative shrinking of the cerebral white matter, which now can be seen as a discrete hyperintense band between the cortex and the intermediate zone. Discrete basal ganglia are not yet seen well.

At 22 to 24 weeks, the Sylvian fissures are well seen and show progressive "squaring" at their anterior and posterior margins (Fig. 2). The germinal matrices have relatively decreased in size and are mainly seen around the position of the ganglionic eminences and the lateral walls of the lateral ventricles. The cell sparse zones have diminished in size under the cerebral cortex. Early sulci form in the anteromedial and posterolateral temporal lobes. The parietooccipital, calcarine, cingulate and hippocampal sulci should all be visible or nearly visible by age 24 weeks, whereas the marginal, central, precentral, and collateral sulci; superior frontal sulcus; posterior part of the superior temporal sulcus; interparietal sulci; and posterior opercula should be visible by 27 to 28 weeks.

By 28 weeks (Fig. 3), brain images have a much more familiar appearance. The corpus callosum is thin but has a mature length, Sylvian fissures are easily recognized, and multiple (rather broad) gyri and (rather shallow) sulci are present. From this point until term, more sulci form and extend more deeply into the white matter. After 30 weeks, myelination may be seen on T1 images, mainly in the brain stem and basal ganglia; at about 38 weeks the initial myelin is seen as a small focus of signal change in the posterior limb of the internal capsule.

THE POSTTERM NEONATAL BRAIN
White Matter Myelination

The processes of myelination, sulcation, and establishment (or strengthening) of white matter pathways continue long after birth; indeed, nearly every new repetitive activity of humans alters both axonal connectivity and myelination. However, general milestones have been established for postterm neonatal brain development. At University of California, San Francisco, the authors rely mainly on T1- and T2-weighted images to assess parenchymal myelination at these ages, as the milestones for normal development are well established.

The immediate newborn brain shows several regional changes related to myelination. On T1-weighted images (Fig. 4A, B), myelin is manifested as hyperintensity[2]; specifically, this T1 hyperintensity is seen in the dorsal pons, the decussation of the superior cerebellar peduncles (in the midbrain), the ventrolateral thalami, the posterior limbs of the internal capsules (at the level of, and immediately above, the ventrolateral thalami), and the corticospinal tracts in the centra semiovale. On T2-weighted images (Fig. 4C–F), hypointensity is seen in the dorsal pons, in the midbrain oculomotor nerve nuclei, in the cerebrum at the ventrolateral thalamic nuclei, and in the posterior limbs of the internal capsules. Hypointensity is also seen ventral to the frontal horns of the lateral ventricles, but this represents a tract of migrating neurons en route to the olfactory sulcus,[2,3] rather than myelin.

By age 4 months, MR shows significant progress of the myelination process, with changes seen earlier on T1 images than on T2-weighted images.[4–6] T1 images (Fig. 5A–C) show hyperintensity in the brain stem, middle cerebellar peduncles, cerebral peduncles, anterior and posterior limbs of the internal capsules, along the lateral walls of the temporal horns, trigones and occipital horns of the lateral ventricles, and in the sensory and motor pathways up to the pre- and

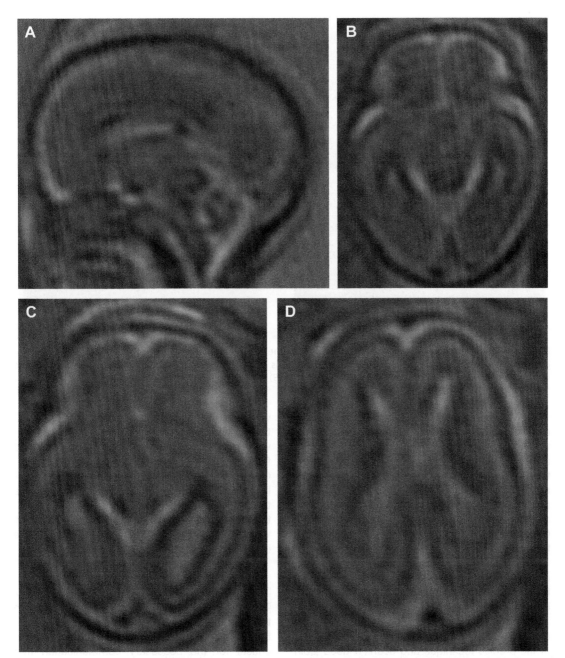

Fig. 1. MR imaging of an 18-week fetal brain. Note the small size of the cerebellar vermis (*A*) and thin layer of white matter between the germinal zone and cortex (*B–D*). Sylvian fissures are barely noticeable.

postcentral gyri. Change is slower on T2-weighted images (Fig. 5D–F), where little change is seen since the neonatal period.[7] The hippocampal commissure shows changes of myelination at this age but not the callosal splenium (Fig. 6).

At age 6 months, further progression of myelination is seen on T1 images (Fig. 7A–D) with hyperintensity extending to the genu of the corpus callosum (see Fig. 7C) and throughout much of the centra semiovale (see Fig. 7D), the areas of exception being the more anterior and basal regions of the frontal lobes and the inferolateral temporal lobes. Changes are seen on the T2-weighted images, as well (Fig. 7E–H), most prominently manifested as increased hypointensity in the motor and, to a lesser extent, in the sensorimotor pathways. Myelination in the corpus callosum remains heterogeneous (Fig. 7I).

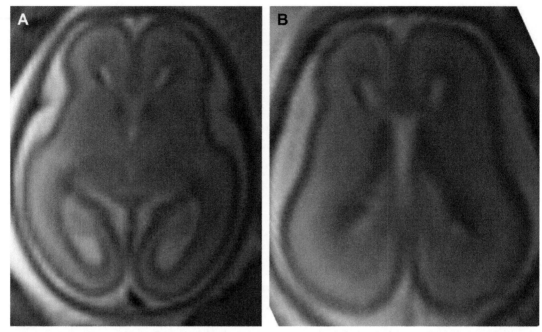

Fig. 2. MR imaging of a 22-week fetal brain. Note that the Sylvian fissures are now well seen (*A*) and show progressive "squaring" at their anterior and posterior margins. The multilayer pattern of the cerebral mantle is more defined with discrete subplate and intermediate zones (*B*). The germinal zone is less prominent.

By age 8 months, T1-weighted images show extensive white matter hyperintensity in most of the cerebrum; the areas of exception being the subcortical white matter of the most rostral portions of the frontal lobes (Fig. 8A, B). On fast spin echo T2-weighted images, significantly more myelin-associated hypointensity is seen in the anterior corpus callosum and in the sensorimotor (precentral and postcentral gyrus) pathways of the cerebrum (Fig. 8C–F).

Beyond the age of about 8 to 10 months, little change is seen on T1-weighted images. However, the hypointensity seen on T2 images progresses, in both the intensity of the (T1 hyperintense and T2 hypointense) signal and the anatomic extent, month by month, with the magnitude likely a result of the precise technique and scanner used (spin echo, fast spin echo, gradient echo, manufacturer, field strength, gradient strength, etc.). As a general rule, the white matter will be nearly completely T2 hypointense by age 20 months and completely T2 hypointense (other than some residual hyperintensity in the areas immediately superolateral to the trigones) by 24 to 26 months (Fig. 9).[2] Tables with detailed description of myelination milestones are available elsewhere and are beyond the scope of this article.[8]

Several investigators have attempted to quantify myelination through the use of several MR imaging techniques, including the ratio of T1-weighted/T2-weighted intensities,[9,10] myelin water fractions,[6] T1 relaxation times,[6] and partial-volume corrected myelin density maps calculated from ratios of T1- and T2-weighted images.[11] Overall, the T1-weighted/T2-weighted maps using a partial volume correction[11] seem to give the best, most reproducible, estimate of myelination; this technique shows that the ratio increases with age between 18 and 35 years, primarily in the innermost cortical layers.[11]

The Corpus Callosum

The corpus callosum is the main bridge between the 2 cerebral hemispheres. It is composed of multiple axons originating in both hemispheres and is critical for the necessary communication that allows the 2 cerebral hemispheres to function in synchrony for most human activities.[12,13] The connections between the 2 hemispheres that allow their necessary communication begin early in development, when axons start to cross the midline after the interhemispheric fissure has formed; the fissure is then remodeled by astroglia from both cerebral hemispheres.[14] The earliest pioneer axons cross at approximately 12 gestational weeks, and most callosal components are present by about 20 weeks,[15] but the corpus continues to grow throughout gestation and childhood: from 20 weeks until term, the callosal

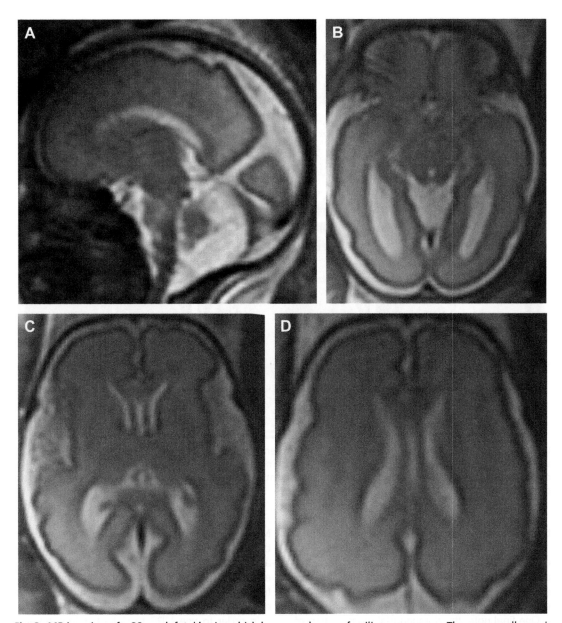

Fig. 3. MR imaging of a 28-week fetal brain, which has a much more familiar appearance. The corpus callosum is of mature length, albeit thin (*A*). Multiple broad gyri and shallow sulci are present with Sylvian fissures easily recognized (*B–D*).

length increases by 25%, the thickness of the callosal body by 30%, and the thickness of the genu by 270%.[15] Not surprisingly, the callosal appearance changes, as well. The neonatal corpus callosum is thin, often uniformly so; as the brain matures, and the axons myelinate, the corpus becomes thicker and, in most cases, grows more rounded. The final shape of the corpus callosum varies significantly among individuals, likely related to precisely how the axons cross the interhemispheric fissure and to which portions of the

contralateral hemisphere they ultimately connect; close analysis will show that no 2 look exactly the same. In general, the mature corpus callosum has a large, rounded genu and splenium with a variably sized body and a narrowing of the body (usually in the posterior half and, often, called the "isthmus"). Other than the abnormally small corpus (thin and of normal length, short and of normal thickness, or thin and short), which is presumed to have fewer interhemispheric axons and, therefore, presumably reduces the connectivity

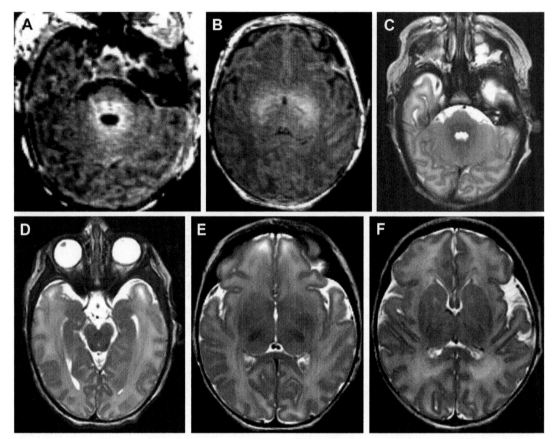

Fig. 4. MR imaging of term neonate. At term T1 hyperintense myelin signal is seen in the dorsal pons (*A*) and in the ventrolateral thalami and posterior limbs of the internal capsules (*B*). T2 hypointense myelin is seen in the dorsal pons (*C*), midbrain oculomotor nerve nuclei (*D*), ventrolateral thalami, and posterior limbs of the internal capsules (*E*, *F*).

between the 2 hemispheres, differences in callosal "morphology" (quotes used because the corpus callosum is not actually a structure, but a collection of individual axons) most often are not associated with any clinical impairment, in the experience of the authors.

One final note: the dorsocaudal most portion of the midline structure known as the corpus callosum is actually the isthmus of the hippocampal commissure; therefore, it myelinates considerably earlier than the remainder of the dorsal corpus callosum (see Fig. 6B). The difference in myelination and the continuity with the fornices can be seen on high-resolution T1 and T2 images.

PROTON MR SPECTROSCOPY

Proton MR spectroscopy (MRS) is an extremely useful tool in assessing brain disease in neonates and infants; its utility continues in childhood when evaluating children with complex disorders that may have a metabolic cause. We acquire

MRS in virtually all encephalopathic neonates because it is easy (and relatively fast) to acquire and, combined with imaging data, it allows differentiation of hypoxic-ischemic encephalopathy from many neonatal and early infantile metabolic encephalopathies.

In order to use MRS to detect pathology, it is essential to understand the appearance of normal neonatal spectra and the evolution of the spectra over the first months of life. The appearance of the MR spectrum varies with the location and the type of acquisition; we almost always acquire long echo time spectra (TE = 270–288 msec) in neonates, because the findings are mainly in N-acetylaspartate (NAA) and lactate, which have long relaxation times. In prematurely born neonates, the long echo spectra show a large choline peak with relatively small creatine and NAA peaks (NAA ranges from about 30% of Cho in the frontal white matter to about 50% in the perirolandic white matter, Figs. 10–12). Small lactate peaks are usually present (see Fig. 11B); these diminish

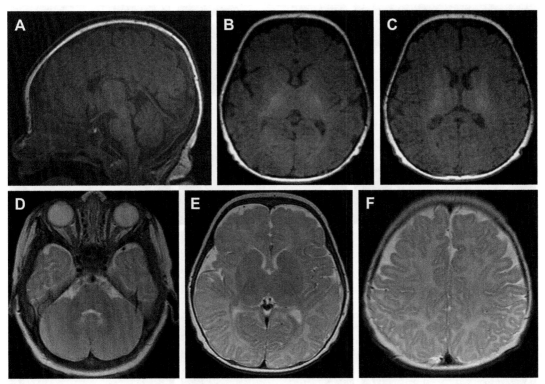

Fig. 5. MR imaging of a 4-month-old infant shows T1 hyperintensity in the brainstem (*A*), anterior and posterior limbs of the internal capsules (*B*) along the trigones of the lateral ventricles (*B*, *C*) and along the sensory and motor pathways (*C*). Little change is seen on T2-weighted images from the neonatal period (*D–F*).

in size as maturation ensues and are rarely seen at birth in the basal ganglia. In the frontal lobes, small lactate peaks can still be found during the first 2 to 3 months after a term birth. After term-equivalent age, the quantity of NAA quickly enlarges compared with other molecular peaks; it becomes dominant compared with other peaks visible on normal spectra by the age of ~6 months and remains so in the absence of degeneration or disease.

Other than looking for decreased area under NAA peaks and increased area under lactate,

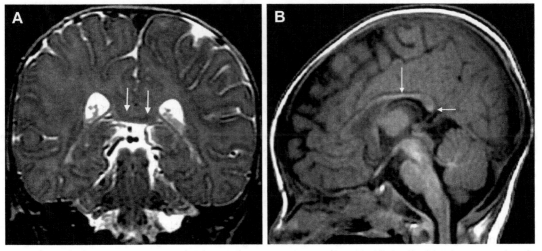

Fig. 6. On this T2-weighted coronal (*A*) T1-weighted sagittal (*B*) images of a 4-month-old infant, note that the hippocampal commissure myelinates before the splenium of the corpus callosum (*arrows*).

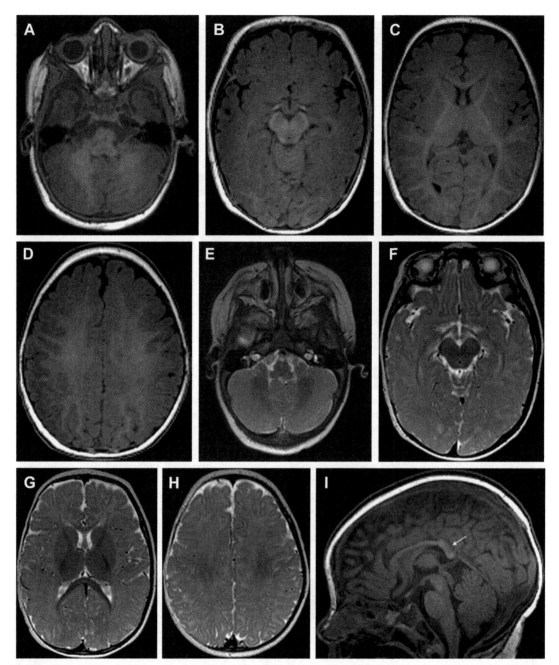

Fig. 7. MR imaging of a 6-month-old infant shows further progression of myelination of T1-weighted images (*A–D*) with hyperintensity of much of the centra semiovale, except the anterior frontal lobe and inferolateral temporal lobes (*B*). On T2-weighted images (*E–H*), increased hypointensity is seen in the internal capsules (*G*) and sensorimotor pathways (*H*). T1 hyperintense myelin extends into the genu of the corpus callosum with a partially myelinated splenium (*arrow*) (*I*). Further progression of myelination is seen on T1 images with hyperintensity extending to the genu of the corpus callosum and throughout much of the centra semiovale, the areas of exception being the more anterior and basal regions of the frontal lobe and the inferolateral temporal lobes. Changes are seen on the T2-weighted images, as well, most prominently manifested as increased hypointensity in the internal capsules (and, to a lesser extent, in the sensorimotor pathways).

long echo spectra are not particularly useful in infants and young children. As most organic compounds have relatively short T2 relaxation times, however, short echo spectra (TE = 20–30 msec) can show the relative concentration of many biologically interesting compounds, such as glutamate and glutamine (peaks at 2.1, 2.4 and 3.75 ppm), myoinositol (peaks at 3.56 and

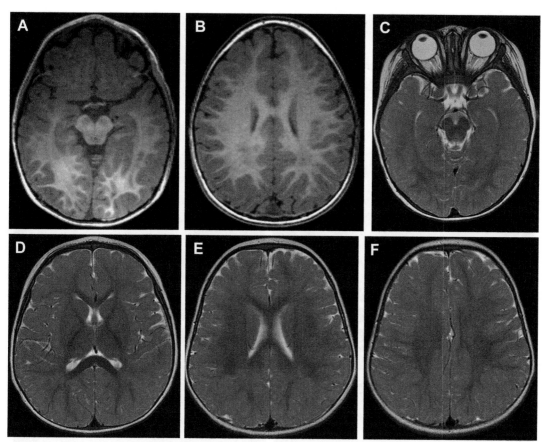

Fig. 8. MR imaging of a 12-month-old child shows near-complete T1 hyperintensity of the cerebral white matter (*A*, *B*) with the exception of the rostral frontal white matter (*A*). On T2-weighted images, more myelin is seen in the sensorimotor pathways of the cerebrum (*C–F*) and in the anterior corpus callosum (*D*, *E*).

4.06 ppm), glucose (at 3.43 ppm), and taurine (2 triplets at 3.2 and 3.42 ppm). All neonates and infants have the so-called "macromolecular peaks;" broad peaks that arise from methyl (at ~0.9 ppm) and methylene (at ~1.3 ppm) are composed of functional groups from many different molecular compounds,[2] thought to largely result from protons in cytosol, the aqueous component of cellular cytoplasm.[16] These are quite prominent on short echo time spectra in infants; they gradually get smaller over the first 12 to 18 months after term and are uncommonly seen after the second birthday.

DIFFUSION IMAGING

MR imaging can be used to measure the rate and direction of the diffusion of water molecules in the brain; this information can be used to assess brain development and to determine whether the development is normal or anomalous. Inside neurons and glia, molecules within and on the surfaces of organelles such as nuclei, mitochondria, ribosomes, etc. increasingly reduce free intracellular water flow as the cell matures; other intracellular organelles, such as endosomes, exosomes, shedding microvesicles, and lysosomes, along with axons navigating through the developing brain, decrease water motion in the extracellular spaces.[17] All of these effects alter the flow patterns of the water molecules (and, thereby, caused reduced or "restricted" diffusion). The largest change in the water motion is likely the result of myelination, in which hydrophobic oligodendrocyte processes extend around the axons coursing throughout the subarachnoid spaces and coat them with a fatty substance (myelin) that repels water. As a result, the water molecules are forced to follow less impeded routes, resulting in highly anisotropic water motion. Although anisotropy (sometimes high levels) can develop before myelination as a result of neurofilament development, changes in intra- and extracellular matrices, aligned axons, single membrane barriers, and cohesive/compact fiber tracts, the development of oligodendrocytes and the subsequent axonal

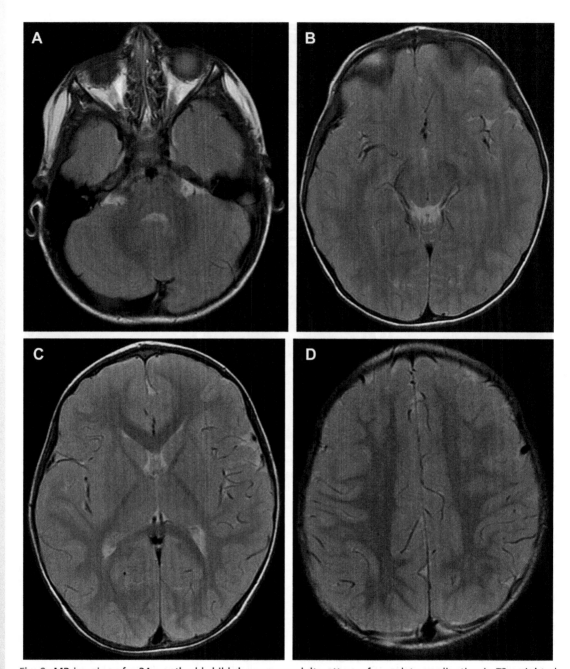

Fig. 9. MR imaging of a 24-month-old child shows near-adult pattern of complete myelination in T2-weighted images (A–D), with only slight residual T2 hyperintensity in the terminal zones adjacent to the trigones of the lateral ventricles (C).

myelination (covering of axons with a hydrophobic coat) seems to be the most important factor in the development of anisotropy.[18,19]

Krogsrud and colleagues[20] showed that during childhood (ages 4–11), there is an overall linear increase in global fractional anisotropy (FA) with decreases in mean diffusivity and radial diffusivity, although the changes of individual tracts are nonlinear for many diffusion tensor imaging

metrics and show regional differences.[20] The rate of change in FA was greater in the left hemisphere, decreased with age, and was greater in frontal regions during this period for all metrics.[20]

RESTING STATE NETWORKS

Resting state functional connectivity MR imaging is a method for investigating the functional

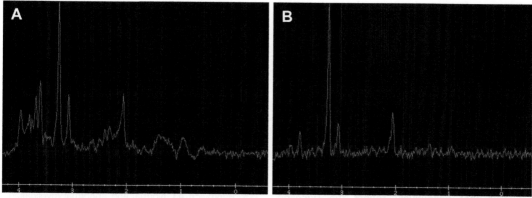

Fig. 10. (*A*) Short (TE = 35 ms) and (*B*) long (TE = 228 ms) echo MRS of a premature neonate (gestational age of 30 weeks) showing the diminished area under the NAA peak (2.0 ppm) relative to the area under the choline peak (3.2 ppm).

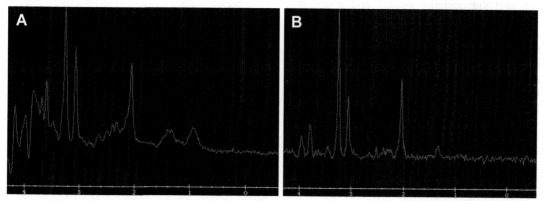

Fig. 11. (*A*) Short (TE = 35 ms) and (*B*) long (TE = 228 ms) echo MRS of a normal term neonate. Note the tiny lactate peak (1.3 ppm), which is normal in a term infant.

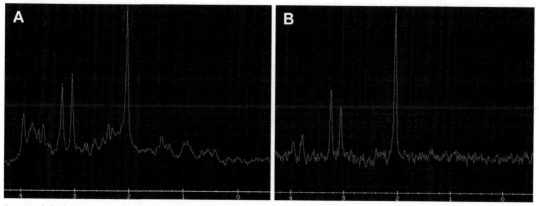

Fig. 12. (*A*) Short (TE = 35 ms) and (*B*) long (TE = 228 ms) echo MRS of a normal child (age 9 years). Note the relatively larger area on the NAA peak (2.0 ppm) relative to the area under the choline peak (3.2 ppm). This pattern is reversed from the premature neonate.

connectivity of the brain by using spontaneous, low-frequency (<0.1 Hz) coherent fluctuations in blood oxygen level–dependent signal to identify networks of functional connections within the cerebrum.[21,22] Resting state networks will likely become an important MR imaging analytical tool in the future; at this time, it is a research tool that may help us to improve our understanding of associations between brain maturation and brain function. Characterization of neural networks using such techniques has improved understanding of the brain's functional topography and led to the discovery of resting state networks (RSN), neural networks that collectively reflect the baseline neuronal activity of the human brain in the absence of goal-directed activities or stimulation.[23] The discovery of the first RSNs led to the discovery of many more: the visual network (spanning much of the occipital cortex); the auditory network (including Heschl gyrus, the superior temporal gyrus, and the posterior insula); and a language network including Broca and Wernicke areas, extending to prefrontal, temporal, parietal, and subcortical regions.[24] Many others are identified, as well, in adults including the thalamus,[25] cerebral cortex,[26] and white matter pathways.[27] Although resting state networks are reasonably well studied in adults, much less in known about them in children. A few studies have attempted to use fMR imaging to identify RSNs in a small number of infants,[21,28] toddlers, children, and adolescents,[29,30] but, because of the small numbers, only rudimentary information was acquired: the default mode network was identified along with RSNs related to attention and executive control.

SUMMARY

Although functional imaging continues to improve and increase our comprehension of the developing brain, anatomic MR imaging remains the primary tool of physicians in assessing normal brain development and in detecting developmental abnormalities, injuries, and metabolic and neoplastic conditions that impair development. The rapid improvements in MR imaging quality and functional MR promise that the future will provide improved diagnoses, built on the fundamentals discussed here.

REFERENCES

1. Lefèvre J, Germanaud D, Dubois J, et al. Are developmental trajectories of cortical folding comparable between cross-sectional datasets of fetuses and preterm newborns? Cereb Cortex 2016;26(7): 3023–35.

2. Barkovich MJ, Barkovich AJ. Normal development of the fetal, neonatal, and infant brain, skull and spine. In: Barkovich AJ, Raybaud C, editors. Pediatric neuroimaging. 6th edition. Philadelphia: Wolters-Kluwer; 2019. p. 18–80.

3. Paredes MF, James D, Gil-Perotin S, et al. Extensive migration of young neurons into the infant human frontal lobe. Science 2016;354(6308):aaf7073.

4. van der Knaap MS. Myelination and myelin disorders: a magnetic resonance study in infants, children and young adults. Utrecht (The Netherlands): Free University of Amsterdam and Universtiy of Utrecht; 1991 [Ph.D.].

5. Barkovich AJ. Normal and abnormal myelination in children. Paper presented at: American Roentgen Ray Society. Orlando, May 3, 1992.

6. Deoni SCL, Dean DC 3rd, Remer J, et al. Cortical maturation and myelination in healthy toddlers and young children. Neuroimage 2015;115:147–61.

7. van der Knaap MS, Valk J. Magnetic resonance of myelin, myelination, and myelin disorders. 2nd edition. Berlin: Springer; 1995.

8. Barkovich AJ, Raybaud C. Pediatric neuroimaging. Philadelphia: Wolters Kluwer Health; 2018.

9. Glasser MF, van Essen DC. Mapping human cortical areas in vivo based on myelin content as revealed by T1- and T2-weighted MRI. J Neurosci 2011;31: 11597–616.

10. Soun JE, Liu MZ, Cauley KA, et al. Evaluation of neonatal brain myelination using the T1- and T2-weighted MRI ratio. J Magn Reson Imaging 2016; 46(3):690–6.

11. Shafee R, Buckner RL, Fischl B. Gray matter myelination of 1555 human brains using partial volume corrected MRI images. Neuroimage 2015;105: 473–85.

12. Huang H, Shu N, Mishra V, et al. Development of human brain structural networks through infancy and childhood. Cereb Cortex 2015;25(5):1389–404.

13. Toga AW, Clark KA, Thompson PM, et al. Mapping the human connectome. Neurosurgery 2012;71(1):1–5.

14. Gobius I, Morcom L, Suarez R, et al. Astroglial-mediated remodeling of the interhemispheric midline is required for the formation of the corpus callosum. Cell Rep 2016;17(3):735–47.

15. Rakic P, Yakovlev PI. Development of the corpus callosum and cavum septae in man. J Comp Neurol 1968;132:45–72.

16. Behar KL, Ogino T. Characterization of macromolecule resonances in the 1H NMR spectrum of rat brain. Magn Reson Med 1993;30(1):38–44.

17. Mathivanan S, Ji H, Simpson RJ. Exosomes: extracellular organelles important in intercellular communication. J Proteomics 2010;73(10):1907–20.

18. Beaulieu C. The basis of anisotropic water diffusion in the nervous system – a technical review. NMR Biomed 2002;15:435–55.

19. Drobyshevsky A, Song S-K, Gamkrelidze G, et al. Developmental changes in diffusion anisotropy coincide with immature oligodendrocyte progression and maturation of compound action potential. J Neurosci 2005;25:5988–97.

20. Krogsrud SK, Fjell AM, Tamnes CK, et al. Changes in white matter microstructure in the developing brain—a longitudinal diffusion tensor imaging study of children from 4 to 11 years of age. Neuroimage 2016;124(Pt A):473–86.

21. Smyser CD, Snyder AZ, Neil JJ. Functional connectivity MRI in infants: exploration of the functional organization of the developing brain. Neuroimage 2011;56(3):1437–52.

22. Biswal B, Yetkin FZ, Haughton VM, et al. Functional connectivity in the motor cortex of resting human brain using echo-planar MRI. Magn Reson Med 1995;34(4):537–41.

23. Fox MD, Raichle ME. Spontaneous fluctuations in brain activity observed with functional magnetic resonance imaging. Nat Rev Neurosci 2007;8:700.

24. Lee MH, Smyser CD, Shimony JS. Resting-state fMRI: a review of methods and clinical applications. Am J Neuroradiol 2013;34(10):1866.

25. Hwang K, Bertolero MA, Liu WB, et al. The human thalamus is an integrative hub for functional brain networks. J Neurosci 2017;37(23):5594–607.

26. Park H-J, Friston K. Structural and functional brain networks: from connections to cognition. Science 2013;342(6158):1238411.

27. Peer M, Nitzan M, Bick AS, et al. Evidence for functional networks within the human brain's white matter. J Neurosci 2017;37(27):6394.

28. Fransson P, Åden U, Blennow M, et al. The functional architecture of the infant brain as revealed by resting-state fMRI. Cereb Cortex 2011;21(1):145–54.

29. Gao W, Zhu H, Giovanello KS, et al. Evidence on the emergence of the brain's default network from 2-week-old to 2-year-old healthy pediatric subjects. Proc Natl Acad Sci U S A 2009;106(16):6790–5.

30. Fair DA, Cohen AL, Dosenbach NUF, et al. The maturing architecture of the brain's default network. Proc Natl Acad Sci U S A 2008;105(10):4028–32.

Ultrasound and MR Imaging of the Normal Fetal Brain

Beth M. Kline-Fath, MD, FAIUM

KEYWORDS

- Prenatal imaging • Ultrasonography • Fetal MR imaging • Fetal brain

KEY POINTS

- Multiplanar high-quality US and MR imaging are essential for complete evaluation of the fetal brain.
- The normal fetal brain changes dramatically intrauterine.
- Knowledge of the US and MR imaging appearance of the normal fetal brain throughout pregnancy is essential for accurate interpretation of normal and abnormal.

INTRODUCTION

Imaging the fetal brain is imaging embryology. Understanding normal brain development is essential because the fetal brain changes dramatically during pregnancy. To define a brain malformation, one must be careful not to misinterpret normal development as abnormal. This article reviews ultrasound (US) and MR imaging of the normal fetal brain anatomy in the second and third trimesters. Biometry of the fetal brain is necessary to verify normal growth; however, standard measurements via gestational age, are not provided herein.

IMAGING

Ultrasonography

Indications/safety

US is the mainstay of pregnancy and fetal imaging, given that it is noninvasive, lacks ionizing radiation, has widespread availability, and real-time and color Doppler capabilities. It is safe, using standard guidelines for obstetric scanning (Box 1).[1]

Gestational age

US can be obtained throughout the second and third trimester, as early as 12 weeks, but most examinations are performed mid gestation at around 20 weeks.

Technique

Transducer selection is determined by maternal body habitus and fetal head positioning. The highest-frequency transducer is typically selected because it provides better spatial resolution but at the expense of decreased sound penetration. Most neurosonography examinations are performed with a 3- to 5-MHz transabdominal transducer or a 5- to 10-MHz transvaginal probe.[2]

Three axial standard (Fig. 1) views allow brain biometry measurements and identification of important fetal brain landmarks (Box 2).[2,3]

Color and power Doppler can define cerebral vascular anatomy (Fig. 2).

Sagittal and coronal imaging of the fetal brain can be obtained transabdominally using a transfontanelle approach, transvaginal when the fetal head is vertex, and/or with 3D imaging.[3] Four coronal images including transfrontal, transcaudate, transthalamic, and transcerebellar (Fig. 3), and 3 sagittal planes, midline and bilateral parasagittal (Fig. 4), should be obtained.[2]

3D imaging allows multiplanar reformats and can be obtained in 98% of second trimester

No disclosures for conflict of interest.
Department of Radiology, Cincinnati Children's Hospital Medical Center, 3333 Burnet Avenue, Cincinnati, OH 45229, USA
E-mail address: beth.kline-fath@cchmc.org

Neuroimag Clin N Am 29 (2019) 339–356
https://doi.org/10.1016/j.nic.2019.03.001
1052-5149/19/© 2019 Elsevier Inc. All rights reserved.

neuroimaging.theclinics.com

sonographic examinations.[3,4] Slice thickness can be increased to obtain a 2D image with more contrast and depth.[3] 3D techniques that may prove helpful include sonoangiography, using the inversion mode, which displays cerebrospinal fluid (CSF) spaces echogenically, and surface-rendering techniques that can provide details of the face or cranium (**Fig. 5**). Using 2D and 3D techniques, neurosonographic examinations have been reported to establish diagnosis in 83.7% of studies in which

a central nervous system malformation is present.[5]

Limitations are listed in **Table 1**.

MR imaging

Indications/safety

Fetal MR imaging is usually performed after identification of an anomaly on prenatal US but may be performed if there is a familial genetic syndrome or a known disorder that predisposes the fetus to harm. MR imaging complements US by providing multiplanar capabilities, large field of view, superior soft tissue contrast, and high resolution. Both sides of the fetal brain and posterior fossa anatomy can be evaluated without artifact from calvarial ossification. MR imaging is less affected by amniotic fluid deficiency or maternal obesity. Griffiths and colleagues[6] recently demonstrated that, in fetuses with abnormal US and brain malformations, MR imaging provided additional diagnostic information in 50%, changed prognostic

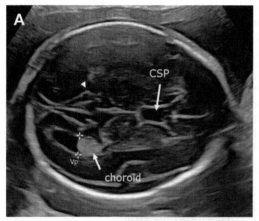
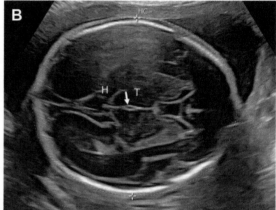
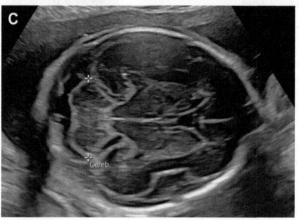

Fig. 1. Standard axial US images of the fetal brain at 24 weeks. (*A*) Transventricular with measurement of atrium of the lateral ventricle with CSP and choroid. The arrowhead demarcates the occipito-parietal sulcus. (*B*) Transthalamic with head circumference measurement. T, thalamus; H, hippocampus, and the arrow depicts the third ventricle. (*C*) Transcerebellar with transverse cerebellum measurement. CSP, cavum septum pellucidum.

Box 2
US standard axial views with anatomy and biometry

- Transventricular:
  - Anatomy: CSP, frontal and posterior horns of LVs containing choroid plexus.
  - Biometry: LV size.
- Transthalamic:
  - Anatomy: frontal horn LV, CSP, thalami, hippocampal gyri.
  - Biometry: head circumference, biparietal and occipitofrontal diameter.
- Transcerebellar:
  - Anatomy: frontal horn LV, CSP, thalami, cerebellum, cisterna magna.
  - Biometry: transcerebellar diameter, cisterna magna.

Abbreviations: CSP, cavum septum pellucidum; LV, lateral ventricles.

information in 20%, and clinical management in more than one-third of cases.

MR imaging safety concerns in pregnancy are primarily with regard to potential teratogenic effects, with highest risk in the first trimester. Heat production, monitored by specific absorption rate, occurs during MR imaging. The question is whether heat will have an effect on developing human cells.[7] In a recent study in which pregnant women in the first trimester were exposed to MR imaging for maternal indications, no negative effects to the fetus were found.[8] Although fetal MR imaging does not yet have Food and Drug Administration approval, American College of Radiology guidelines state that fetal MR imaging should be performed when the benefits outweigh the risks.[9] MR imaging contrast should not be administered because gadolinium crosses the placenta, and a recent study showed deleterious effects, including increased risk for stillbirth and neonatal death.[7,8]

Gestational age
Most MR examinations are performed in the second and third trimester, typically after 18 weeks gestation, due to teratogenic risks and fetal size limitations.

Technique
MR imaging can be performed at 1.5T or 3T. Imaging at 1.5T is easier because 3T has propensity for higher heat deposition and artifacts, the most distracting being blackout in the center of the imaging.[7] However, high field strength improves image resolution, and there is evidence that 3T imaging may provide better central nervous system anatomic detail.[10]

Fast imaging is essential because sedation is not typically administered. The fetal brain has a high water content; therefore, heavy T2-weighted sequences provide best detail. Performing anatomic imaging is essential for accurate interpretation. Imaging sequences and indications are listed in **Box 3** with images in **Fig. 6**.

Fetal brain measurements verify normal growth.[11] The entire fetus should be evaluated because anomalies in other organs may provide important clues to genetic syndromes.

Limitations are listed in **Table 1**, but, as with US, because image quality is operator dependent the need for education and training must be stressed.

Higher-level MR imaging techniques, including spectroscopy, diffusion tractography, and functionality, require longer acquisition times but can be performed in the fetus. In addition, multiple new post processing techniques, including motion correction, automated tissue delineation, 3D printing, and artificial intelligence are new frontiers in both US and MR imaging, which, because of length constraints, will not be covered.

NORMAL FETAL BRAIN

An organized approach is imperative when evaluating the fetal brain. In this review, anatomy via US and MR imaging is presented central to peripheral, beginning with the ventricles.

Ventricles

Lateral ventricles
The lateral ventricles (LVs) change dramatically. Before 16 weeks, the LVs are globular and large, filled with choroid plexus. With growth of the

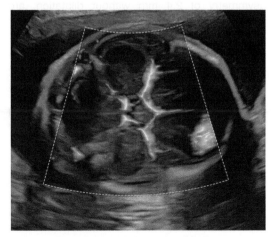

Fig. 2. Color Doppler of the circle of Willis.

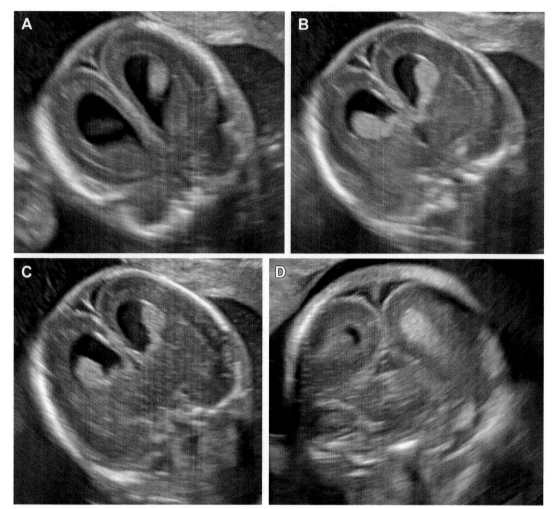

Fig. 3. Normal 17 week transvaginal coronal US (*A*), transfrontal (*B*), transcaudate (*C*), transthalamic, and (*D*) transcerebellar

corpus callosum (CC), basal ganglia (BG), periventricular white matter, and frontal and occipital lobes, the LV narrows, achieving a smaller adult-like configuration. The walls of the ventricle should be smooth. The atrial diameter is relatively constant from 14 to 40 weeks, with normal values being less than 10 mm.[12]

Ultrasonography The LVs are anechoic, containing an echogenic choroid plexus. The measurement of LVs on a transventricular plane should be at the level of the parieto-occipital sulcus and glomus of the choroid plexus, with the calipers placed in the largest part of the atrium inside the echogenic interface, which defines the LV walls (see **Fig. 1**A). A coronal image at the level of the atria can be used if axial plane imaging is not possible. The normal mean diameter of the atrium of the lateral ventricle is 7.6 ± 0.6 mm from 14 to

38 weeks.[13] Separation of ≤3 mm between the choroid plexus and wall of the LV, and ventricular asymmetry of 2.4 mm without dilatation, are considered normal.[14]

MR imaging Similar to US, the LVs can be measured on the axial plane at the level of the thalamus, with average normal values being 6 to 7 mm, discrepant with US by 1 to 2 mm, and threshold for ventriculomegaly greater than 10 mm[15] Coronal measurements inside the atrial wall at the level of the choroid plexus are favored because they are highly concordant with US (**Fig. 7**).[16]

Cavum septum pellucidum
The cavum septum pellucidum (CSP) is closely associated to development of the CC. It is an important space lined by 2 thin membranes that extend from the anterior part of the CC, inferior

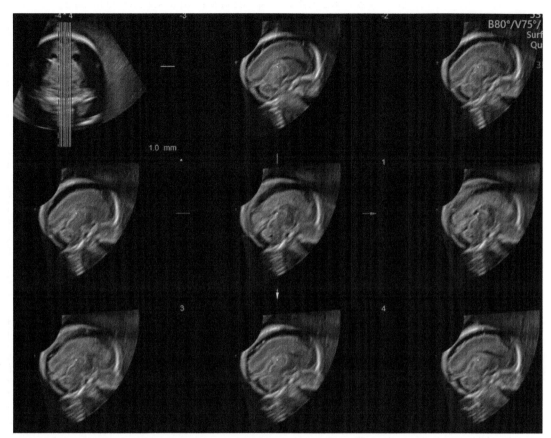

Fig. 4. Sagittal 3D US midline/paramidline in a 17-week fetus.

to the surface of the fornix and lateral along inner walls of the LV. The cavum septum vergae (CSV) is posterior to CSP. The CSP can be visualized as early as 15 weeks, but should be present by 18 weeks gestation.[17] CSP will increase in size to approximately 27 weeks, with normal diameter between 2 and 10 mm.[18] CSV will fuse by 40 weeks, and CSP as early as 37 weeks, but typically postnatal between 3 to 6 months of age.[17,18]

Ultrasonography The CSP is an anechoic rectangular CSF space between the anterior horns of the LVs (see **Fig. 1A**).[2] The inferior hypoechoic columns of the fornix containing central linear echogenicity should not be confused with the CSP (**Fig. 8**).

MR imaging The CSP is a cystic space lined by 2 parallel intermediate T2 signal leaflets (**Fig. 9**).

Third ventricle, aqueduct of Sylvius, and fourth ventricle
The third ventricle is a linear single echogenic line early in the second trimester, subsequently seen as parallel echogenic lines (see **Fig. 1B**) on US.[19] Using MR imaging, the third ventricle is a linear CSF space, best depicted on axial or coronal

imaging (see **Fig. 9**). The size is relatively stable, with maximum transverse dimension less than 4 mm.[19,20]

The aqueduct of Sylvius is a thin linear CSF space between the midbrain and tectum, which is suggested on sagittal midline US (**Fig. 10**), but is better depicted on MR imaging (**Fig. 11**).

The fourth ventricle is apparent between 5 and 7 weeks owing to development of a large CSF cavity termed Blake's pouch. This structure disappears in the first trimester, leaving the fourth ventricle as a triangular CSF space. On US, the fourth ventricle is apparent in 89% of transabdominal images and 100% of transvaginal images (see **Fig. 11**), with axial anterior to posterior dimensions at 3.5 ± 1.3 mm.[21] On MR imaging, using the sagittal plane (see **Fig. 11**), the fourth ventricle should measure, from the dorsal pons to the fastigial point, 4.5 + 2.5 mm, with a maximum dimension less than 7 mm.[20]

Parenchyma

Supratentorial
The germinal matrix (GM), which includes the ventricular zone (VZ) and subventricular zone (SVZ), is

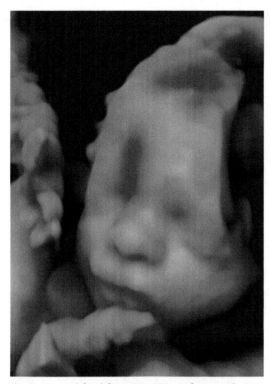

Fig. 5. Normal fetal face using 3D surface rendering.

Box 3
Standard fetal brain MR imaging sequences and indications

1. Single-shot rapid acquisition with refocused echoes (SS-RARE or SSFSE)

   Best brain parenchymal detail

2. True fast imaging with steady-state free precession (SSFP)

   Midline brain, sulcation, bright blood

3. Cine SSFP

   Fetal swallowing/movement

4. Diffusion

   Ischemia

   Myelination

   T2* image for hemorrhagic products

5. T1-weighted/multiplanar spoiled gradient recall acquisition in steady state (FMSPRGR)

   Hemorrhage, fat, calcification

   Myelination

   Pituitary gland

6. Gradient echo T2

   Hemorrhage

the origin of cerebral/cortical cells and lies along the walls of the ventricular system. The volume increases exponentially to 23 weeks; with one-half of the volume lost from 26 to 28 weeks.[22] The VZ, along the ependyma early in fetal life, provides direct descendants of the neural plate and gives rise to the SVZ, located subependymal to the fetal white matter. SVZ is an important source of cortical and striatal neurons, astrocytes, and glial cells. Ganglionic eminence (GE) within the SVZ is present at the caudothalamic groove and adjacent to the atrium of the lateral ventricle. These areas are focally thick because of the high cell density and give rise to the deep gray nuclei, thalamus, and glial cells. Within the SVZ, deep to the white matter, is a cell-sparse area known as the periventricular rich zone (PVRZ), where axons of the CC develop. The central white matter, known as the intermediate zone (IZ), increases dramatically in size during gestation with migrating glial and neuronal cells passing through the area to reach their final destination. From 20 to 30 weeks, the periventricular crossroads (PVCs), which represents developing, intersecting white matter tracts, are noted adjacent to the frontal, atrial, and temporal horns, and retrolenticular internal capsule.[23] Intrauterine until approximately 32 to 34 weeks, the fetal cortex contains 7 layers, with the deepest representing the subplate (SP), containing maturing neurons and afferent fibers, important for columnar organization of the final 6-layered cortex. Myelination of the cerebrum is not apparent until late third trimester.

Table 1	
Limitations of prenatal US and MR imaging	
US	**MR imaging**
Operator dependent	Operator dependent
Early imaging limits anomaly detection	Early imaging limits anomaly detection
Small field of view	Small fetal size (<16 wk)
Limited soft tissue contrast	Partial volume averaging
Diminished detail	Diminished detail
Fetal position	Maternal motion
Fetal motion	Fetal motion (polyhydramnios)
Lack of amniotic fluid	Some with low amniotic fluid
Maternal obesity	Mildly with maternal obesity
Acoustic shadowing	Maternal claustrophobia
Artifact brain closest transducer	
≥ 28 wk with calvarial ossification	

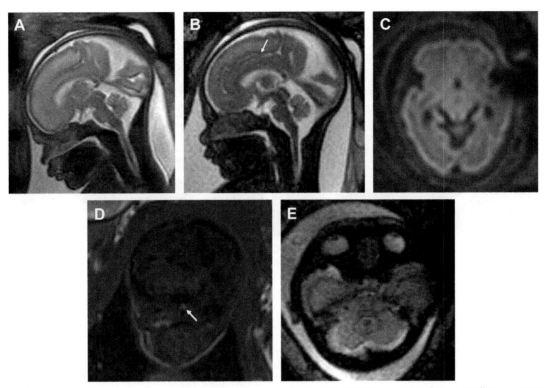

Fig. 6. Routine MR imaging sequences in a 29-week fetus. (A) Sagittal SSFSE T2 image shows excellent contrast and resolution resulting in high parenchymal detail. (B) Sagittal SSFP T2 image accentuates water and soft tissue interfaces (*white arrow* cingulate sulcus). (C) Axial diffusion at the level of the cerebral peduncles. (D) Coronal T1 imaging with hyperintense pituitary (*arrow*). (E) Axial gradient echo posterior fossa.

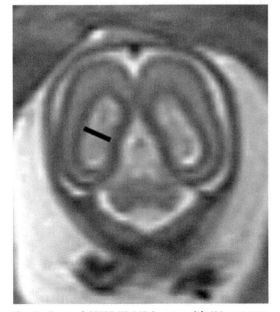

Fig. 7. Coronal SSFSE T2 MR image with LV measurements (*black line*) inside the atrial wall.

Lamination

Ultrasonography The surface of the brain demonstrates increased echogenicity because of the presence of pia and sulci, and the brain parenchyma is hypoechoic. Between 17 and 28 weeks, the cortical plate and SP are hypoechoic and indistinguishable, and the IZ demonstrates mild increased echogenicity allowing for identification of an SP-IZ interface (Fig. 12).[24] The GM may be seen as a narrow smooth zone of increased echogenicity along the ventricular wall from 17 to 28 weeks; however, depiction of the GM is difficult on routine sonography.

MR imaging The lamination pattern changes depending on gestational age.[25,26] The cortex and GM along the walls of the LVs demonstrates high cellularity, represented by T1 and T2 shortening. The early IZ lacks myelination, and is high in water content, demonstrating T1 and T2 prolongation. The PVRZ and SP, because of the high extracellular matrix, also demonstrates T1 and T2 prolongation. Areas of high cellularity, including GM and cortex, show high signal on diffusion and low signal on the apparent diffusion coefficient

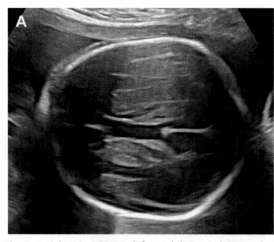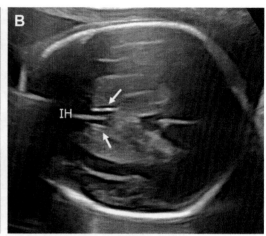

Fig. 8. Axial US in a 25-week fetus. (*A*) Normal CSP and CSV. (*B*) Inferior are the columns of the fornix mimicking a CSP (*arrows*). Echogenic midline is the interhemispheric (IH) fissure.

map.[27] The IZ and SP show low signal on diffusion (**Fig. 13**).

16 to 20 weeks Likely due to limited spatial resolution, the fetal brain demonstrates a 3-layered pattern (**Fig. 14**).[25]

> GM: dark T2
> IZ: bright T2
> Cortex: dark T2

The GM will be thick owing to incomplete migration of cells, and the cortex thin owing to incomplete neuronal migration. The GEs will be thick and accentuated and should not be confused with hemorrhage. The BG are homogeneous with white matter, although T2 hyperintensity in the superior thalamus can be depicted (**Fig. 15**).[11]

20 to 30 weeks A time of neuronal migration and organization, the PVRZ and SP are present, and the IZ is more cellular owing to migrating glia, astrocytes, and neurons, resulting in a 5-layered pattern (**Fig. 16**).

> GM: dark T2.
> PVRZ: bright T2.
> IZ: vague dark T2; PVCs focal bright T2.
> SP: bright T2.
> Cortex: dark T2.

After 28 weeks, the GM decreases in size, cortex increases in thickness, IZ increases in T2 signal, and the SP disappears, persisting longest at 30 to 32 weeks in the frontal and anterior

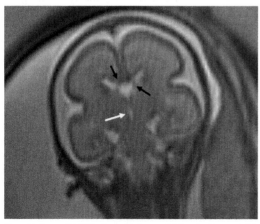

Fig. 9. Coronal MR image in a 25-week fetus with black arrows depicting leaflets of CSP and the white arrow the third ventricle.

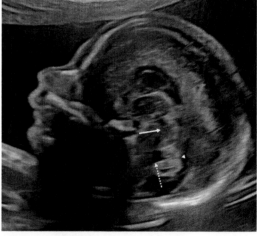

Fig. 10. Sagittal US in a 21-week fetus. The solid arrow points to the aqueduct of Sylvius and the dotted arrow to the fourth ventricle. The primary fissure is demarcated by the arrowhead.

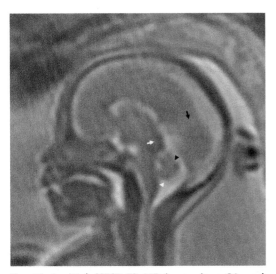

Fig. 11. Sagittal SSFSE T2 MR image in a 21-week fetus. The solid white arrow indicates the aqueduct of Sylvius. Fourth ventricle with sharp posterior recess (fastigial point) noted. The black arrow defines the parieto-occipital sulcus. The vermis with a primary fissure (*black arrowhead*) covers the fourth ventricle. The brainstem is homogeneous, except for the dark signal along the dorsal medulla showing early myelination (*white arrowhead*).

temporal lobes. The deep gray matter, after 26 weeks, demonstrates T2 hypointensity (**Fig. 17**).

30 to 40 weeks The pattern is 2 to 3 layers: being 3-layered in areas with persistent GM,

present in the caudal GE until 33 weeks, and adjacent to the caudate heads to approximately 36 weeks (see **Fig. 17**). Small quantities of pluripotent GM cells persist along the frontal horns postnatally. After 32 weeks, myelination can be seen in the putamen, ventro-lateral thalamus, and posterior limb of the internal.

Sulcation
Cortical sulcation is one of the most accurate ways to date a pregnancy and confirm normal brain development. The Sylvian fissure is the first fissure after the interhemispheric, and begins as a smooth wide vertical indentation, which, with opercularization, greater in the temporal and parietal than frontal insular area, will become angular and then more horizontal with increased sulcation. In the second half of pregnancy, the primary sulci begin developing, initially as a small undulation in the cortex, which then deepens to become V shaped. From the 24th week, secondary sulci will branch from the primary, and then, from 28 weeks, tertiary will arise along the secondary resulting in complex sulcation late in the third trimester. Sulcation by imaging is delayed with regard to the neuropathologic model, as much as 4 to 6 weeks with US and on average 1 to 2 weeks with MR imaging.[28,29] Normal cortical sulcation can be asymmetric on US and MR imaging, with one example being that the right superior temporal gyrus may appear before the left.[30,31]

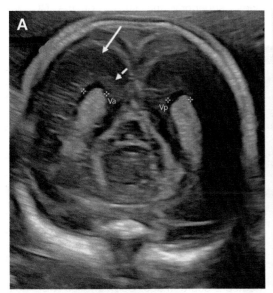
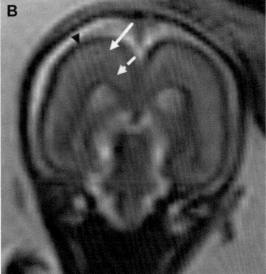

Fig. 12. US and MR imaging of a 23-week fetus. (*A*) Transvaginal coronal US image demonstrates the cortex and SP as hypoechoic (*solid arrow*) and the IZ as mildly echogenic (*dashed arrow*). (*B*) Coronal MR imaging in same fetus showing the cortex (*black arrowhead*), SP (*solid arrow*), and IZ (*dashed arrow*).

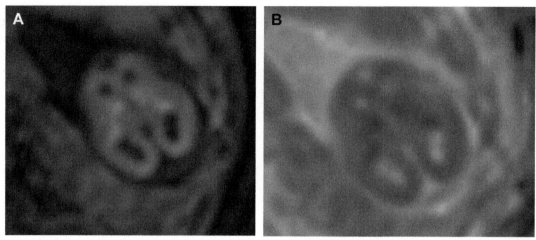

Fig. 13. Diffusion (*A*) and corresponding apparent diffusion coefficient (ADC) (*B*) in a 17-week fetus. Notice that the GEs shows hyperintense diffusion and hypointense ADC.

Ultrasonography Sulci appear as linear bright echoes (**Fig. 18**), seen better along the medial surface than outer brain convexity.[29] Cortical sulci should be imaged perpendicular to the expected sulcus course; however, 30% to 32% of the sulci are not well delineated using the transabdominal approach.[31] Transvaginal and 3D US allow easier depiction of the sulcus. The Sylvian fissure can be defined as early as 14 weeks, with opercularization at 22 to 24 weeks, and coverage by 28 to 35 weeks.[31] Ultrasonography sulci milestones are listed in **Table 2**.[32]

MR imaging MR imaging is excellent at depicting the fetal sulcation (**Figs. 6B, 11,** and **19;** Table 2).[28,33] There can be a delay of 2 weeks from the time the sulcus is identified on MR imaging to when it is present in 75% of fetuses.[33]

Corpus Callosum
The CC is the largest commissure, developing bidirectionally, from 8 to 20 weeks, from the area of the anterior body. The CC has 4 parts: rostrum, genu, body, and splenium.

US The CC is best visualized from the sagittal plane, after 16 weeks, as a thin hypoechoic to anechoic structure bordered by echogenic lines, superiorly the sulcus of the CC and

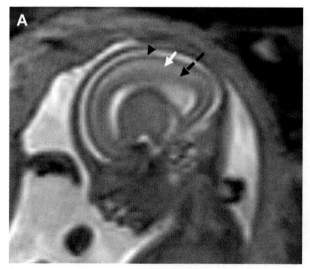
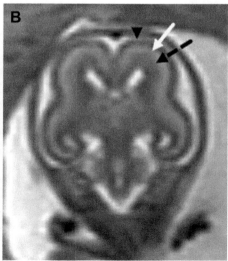

Fig. 14. Sagittal (*A*) and coronal (*B*) SSFSE T2 MR images in a 19-week fetus with 3 layered pattern. Cortex (*arrowhead*), IZ (*solid arrow*), and GM (*dotted arrow*).

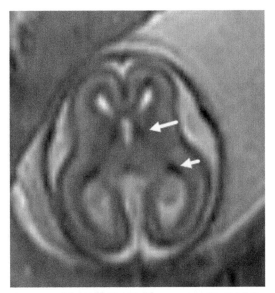

Fig. 15. Axial SSFSE T2 MR image at the level of the superior thalami which demonstrate T2 hyperintensity. The GEs are focally dark T2 signal (*arrows*).

cingulate gyrus, and inferiorly by CSP, CSV, and LV (**Fig. 20A**).[34] 3D imaging can be acquired from the axial plane; however, the technique limits resolution, and the CC is hyperechoic, similar in echogenicity to a lipoma (**Fig. 20B**).[34,35] Sagittal or coronal 3D acquisition provides better detail, because the CC is hypoechoic and allows accurate measurments.[35] Secondary signs for normal development of the CC include the presence of the CSP and normal color Doppler of the pericallosal artery (**Fig. 20C**).[36]

MR imaging The CC is best depicted on a midline sagittal image as a T2 hypointense structure superior to the fornix and should be verified on coronal imaging, inferior to the interhemispheric fissure and superior to the LVs. Before 20 weeks, the CC appears short and horizontal, but demonstrates a more crescentic appearance thereafter (**Fig. 21**). Lack of definition of the rostrum and flexion of the genu, particularly early in gestation, may be difficult, and should not imply abnormality.[37]

Posterior Fossa

The brainstem develops early and matures medulla, pons, and then midbrain. The cerebellum is one of the first brain structures to arise and one of the last to mature, continuing after birth. The cerebellum develops from 2 GM, the VZ along the roof of the fourth ventricle, and the rhombic lips (RLs) laterally at the junction of the roof plate and neural tube. The VZ gives rise to the deep cerebellar nuclei (DCN), Purkinje cells, and interneurons; whereas the RLs provide granule cell precursors and precerebellar nuclei in the brainstem. At the 5th gestational week, with the appearance of the pontine flexure, the primitive cerebellar hemispheres appear followed by the vermis at approximately 9 weeks, which will grow to cover the fourth ventricle by 20 weeks.[38] The development of the cerebellum continues postnatally to result in a 3-layered cerebellar cortex. Myelination occurs first in the dorsal brainstem, progressing from the medulla, through the pons, to the midbrain.

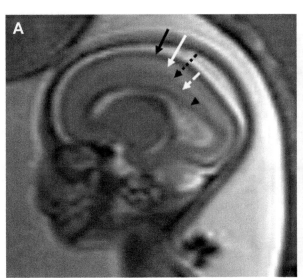
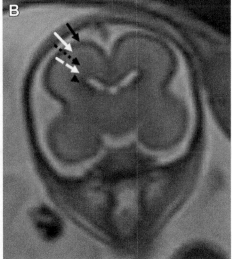

Fig. 16. Sagittal (*A*) and coronal (*B*) SSFSE T2 MR images in a 23-week fetus with 5 layered pattern. Cortex (*black solid arrow*), SP (*white solid arrow*), IZ (*black dotted arrow*), PVRZ (*white dashed arrow*), and GM (*black arrowhead*).

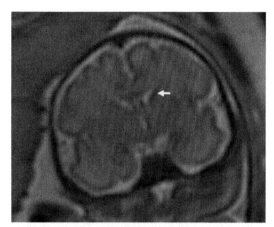

Fig. 17. Coronal SSFSE T2 image in a 33-week fetus. The white arrow depicts residual GM. BG are hypointense.

Lamination

Ultrasonography When evaluating the posterior fossa, multiplanar views are essential. Standard axial imaging shows the cerebellar hemispheres and peduncles and fourth ventricle. The brainstem, cerebellar vermis, fourth ventricle, and tentorium are evaluated by midline sagittal imaging. The brainstem is homogeneous with the pons, showing more echogenicity ventral than dorsal from 21 weeks' gestation onward because of high cellularity and multiple crossing tracts (Fig. 22A).[39]

Cerebellar hemispheres appear homogeneously hypoechoic, and later in gestation with echogenic stripes representing folia (Fig. 22B).

The vermis is more echogenic than the adjacent hemispheres, possibly because of deeper fissures

Table 2
Fetal supratentorial sulcation in weeks detected in 75% of fetuses

Sulcus	US (wk)	MR imaging (wk)
Interhemispheric	18	14–15
Sylvian	18	16–18
Callosal	18	22–23
Parieto-occipital	20	22–23
Hippocampal	18	22–23
Calcarine	22	24–25
Cingulate	24	24–25
Central	28	26
Collateral	—	26
Precentral	30	27
Superior temporal	30	27
Marginal	32	27
Postcentral	30	28
Intraparietal	—	28
Superior frontal	30	29
Inferior frontal	30	29
Inferior temporal	30	33–34
Occipitotemporal	30	33–34

and the interface of arachnoid vessels (see Fig. 22). The inferior vermis is open and communication between the fourth ventricle and cisterna magna (CM) can remain until 18 weeks.[40] After 18 weeks, the vermis should have a brainstem vermian angle of less than 18°.[41]

MR imaging

16 to 20 weeks The brainstem should be homogeneous, with intermediate T2 isointensity, and straight with rounded contours at the level of the pons. The tectum, because of high cellularity, demonstrates T2 hypointensity (see Fig. 21). At 18 weeks, with early myelination, dark T2 signals can been seen in the dorsal medulla (see Fig. 11).

The cerebellum is small and homogeneous with intermediate signals (Fig. 23).[42] The GM is not well defined.

The vermis should cover the fourth ventricle, with accentuation of its most posterior recess, known as the fastigial point, as early as 18 to 20 weeks (see Figs. 11A and 21).[43]

20 to 30 weeks The brainstem continues to grow, showing intermediate T2 signal, but with myelination in the medial longitudinal fasciculus, dark T2 signal is noted dorsal to the level of the pons (Fig. 24A).

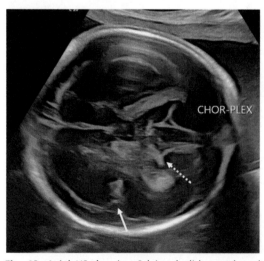

Fig. 18. Axial US showing Sylvian (*solid arrow*) and calcarine (*dotted arrow*) sulcus in a 28-week fetus.

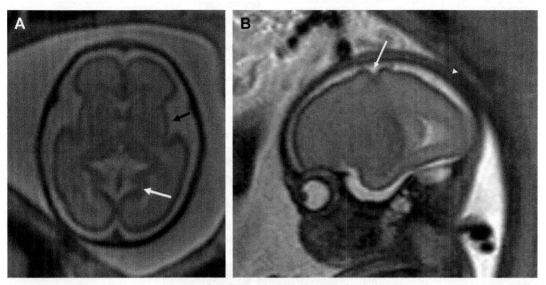

Fig. 19. Coronal (A) and sagittal (B) SSFSE T2 MR images in a 26-week fetus demonstrating normal sulci. (A) Sylvian (*black arrow*) and calcarine sulcus (*white arrow*). (B) Central sulcus (*white arrow*).

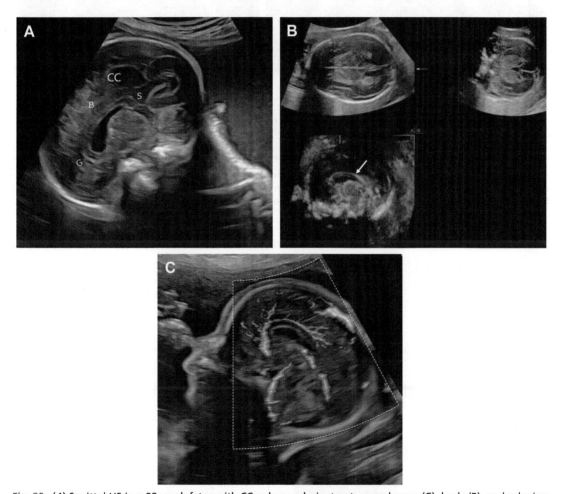

Fig. 20. (A) Sagittal US in a 22-week fetus with CC as hypoechoic structure and genu (G), body (B), and splenium (S) demarcated. (B) 3D axial imaging shows the CC as hyperechoic (*arrow*). (C) Normal color Doppler of the pericallosal artery.

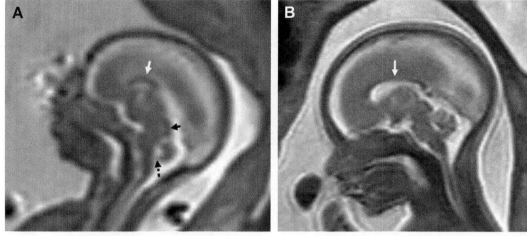

Fig. 21. Sagittal SSFSE T2 MR images. (*A*) Short horizontal CC (*white arrow*) at 17 weeks. Tectum is dark T2 (*black arrow*) and the vermis does not yet cover the fourth ventricle (*dotted arrow*). (*B*) Crescentic CC at 25 weeks (*arrow*).

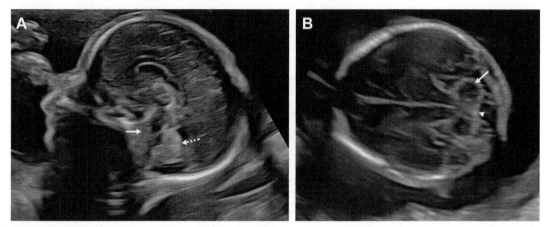

Fig. 22. (*A*) Sagittal US at 24 weeks showing that the brainstem is more echogenic (*solid arrow*) ventral than dorsal. The vermis is echogenic and the primary fissure is seen (*dotted arrow*) (*B*) Axial US at 17 weeks with cerebellar hemispheres hypoechoic (*solid arrow*) and vermis echogenic (*arrowhead*).

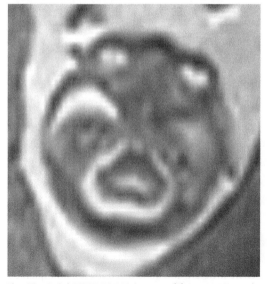

Fig. 23. Axial SSFSE T2 MR image of fetus at 17 weeks with homogeneous cerebellum.

The cerebellum demonstrates a 3-layered pattern (Fig. 24B).[42]

DCN: dark T2
White matter: bright T2
Cortex: dark T2

Table 3		
Fetal infratentorial sulcation in weeks		
	US (wk)	MR imaging (wk)
Primary	18–24	17.5
Prepyramidal	30–32	21
Preculminate	30–32	21–22
Secondary	30–32	24
All vermian	30–32	27
Cerebellar hemisphere	—	24–29

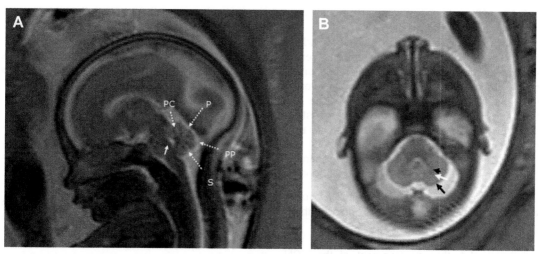

Fig. 24. SSFSE T2 MR images in a 26-week fetus. (*A*) Sagittal imaging shows the homogenous brainstem with myelination to the level of the pons (*solid arrow*). The vermis is parallel to the brainstem and sulcation is complete with the primary (P), prepyramidal (PP), preculminate (PC), and secondary sulci (S) noted. (*B*) Axial image with a 3-layer cerebellum. DCN (*short black arrow*), white matter (*white arrow*), and cortex (*long black arrow*).

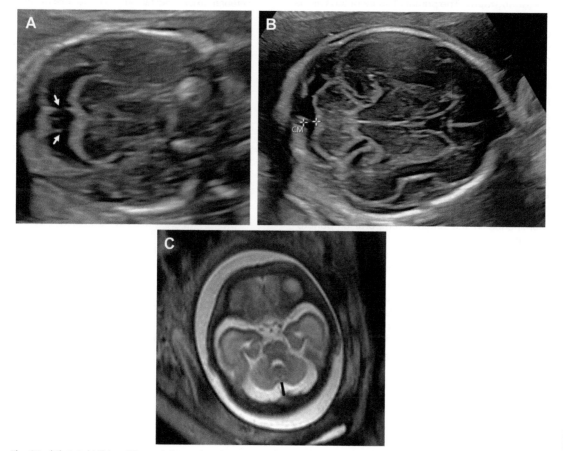

Fig. 25. (*A*) Axial US in a 20-week fetus showing septae (*arrows*) of Blake's pouch. (*B*) Transcerebellar US view with measurements of cisterna magna (CM). (*C*) Axial SSFSE T2 MR image with normal CM measurements.

At 28 to 29 weeks, the inferior and superior cerebellar peduncle are myelinated.[38]

The vermis covers the fourth ventricle, and the angle between the dorsal brainstem and ventral surface of the vermis (tegmento-vermian angle) should be close to 0°.[43] The line in the vermis from the fastigial point to the declive (the folia below the primary fissure) should demonstrate that the tissue inferior (posterior lobe) is larger than the tissue superior (anterior lobe).[43]

After 21 weeks, the tentorium has a definitive orientation perpendicular to the occipital bone.[44]

30 to 40 weeks The brainstem remains T2 hypointense, but myelination reaches the dorsal midbrain and inferior colliculus at 32 weeks.[44]

The cerebellum 3-layer pattern persists. With gyration and further development of the DCN, the central area is T2 hyperintense, with the peripheral gyri T2 hypointense.[44]

Sulcation

The vermis demonstrates sulcation earlier than the cerebellar hemispheres (**Table 3**).[45,46]

Ultrasonography The primary fissure of the vermis can be detected as early as 18 weeks (40%), but uniformly by 24 weeks (see **Figs. 10** and **22**).[45] Differentiation of other fissures are possible by 30 to 32 weeks.

MR imaging The primary fissure is the deepest fissure in the vermis (see **Figs. 11** and **24**A), and the horizontal sulcus for the cerebellar hemispheres.

Subarachnoid Spaces

The spaces appear prominent in the second and early third gestation, but decrease in size from 30 weeks, although there can be mild residual prominence in the anterior temporal or parieto-occipital area.[22]

The cisterna magna (CM) is a septated space, with the septate and medial extent representing Blake's pouch and the lateral cavitation of the meninx primitiva to form subarachnoid space.[46] With US, the septae of the Blake pouch can be delineated (**Fig. 25**A).[46] On MR imaging, the septae are best appreciated on heavy T2 and/or SSFP image. Normal CM measures greater than 2 and less than 10 mm from the vermis to the calvarium on US transcerebellar and MR axial or sagittal image (**Fig. 25**B, C).[46]

SUMMARY

The fetal brain changes throughout gestation, and knowledge of the normal brain and an organized approach is essential. Multiplanar anatomic imaging with US and MR imaging provides the groundwork for accurate assessment. Having a good understanding of embryology is necessary in interpretation of the normal fetal brain.

REFERENCES

1. AIUM-ACR-ACOGG-SMRM-SRU practice parameter for the performance of standard diagnostic obstetric ultrasound examinations. J Ultrasound Med 2018;9999:1–12.

2. Sonographic examination of the fetal central nervous system: guidelines for performing the 'basic examination' and the 'fetal neurosonogram. Ultrasound Obstet Gynecol 2007;29:109–16.

3. Monteagudo A, Timor-Tritsch IE. Normal sonographic development of the central nervous system from the second trimester onwards using 2D, 3D, and transvaginal sonography. Prenat Diagn 2009; 29:326–39.

4. Rizzzo G, Pietrolucci ME, Capece G, et al. Satisfactory rate of post-processing visualization of the fetal cerebral axial, sagittal and coronal planes from three-dimensional volumes acquired in routine second trimester ultrasound practice by sonographers of peripheral centers. J Matern Fetal Neonatal Med 2011;24:1071–6.

5. Paladini D, Quarantelli M, Sglavo G, et al. Accuracy of neurosonography and MRI in clinical mangement of fetuses referred with central nervous system abnormalities. Ultrasound Obstet Gynecol 2014;44: 188–96.

6. Griffiths PD, Bradburn M, Campbell MJ, et al. Use of MRI in the diagnosis of fetal brain abnormalities in utero (MERIDIAN); a multicenter, prospective cohort study. Lancet 2017;389:538–46.

7. Tocchio S, Kline-Fath B, Danal E, et al. MRI evaluation and safety in the developing brain. Semin Perinatol 2015;29(2):73–104.

8. Ray JG, Vermeulen MJ, Bharatha A, et al. Association between MRI exposure during pregnancy and fetal and childhood outcomes. JAMA 2016;316(9): 952–61.

9. Kanal E, Barkovich AJ, Bell C, et al. ACR guidance document on MR safe practices: 2013. J Magn Reson Imaging 2013;37(3):501–30.

10. Priago G, Barrowman NJ, Hurteau-Miller J, et al. Does 3T fetal MRI improve image resolution of the normal brain structures between 20-24 weeks' gestational age? AJNR Am J Neuroradiol 2017;38: 1636–42.

11. Kline-Fath BM. Normal brain imaging. In: Kline-Fath BM, Bulas BI, Bahado-Sing R, editors. Fundamental and advanced fetal imaging. Philadelphia: Wolters Kluwer; 2015. p. P184–219.

12. Farrell TA, Hertzberg BS, Kliewer MA, et al. Fetal lateral ventricles: reassessment of normal values for atrial diameter at US. Radiology 1994;193:409–11.

13. Cardoza JD, Goldstein RB, Filly RA. Exclusion of fetal ventriculomegaly with a single measurement: the width of the lateral ventricular atrium. Radiology 1988;169:711–4.

14. Guibaud L. Fetal cerebral ventricular measurement and ventriculomegaly: time for procedure standardization. Ultrasound Obstet Gynecol 2009;34:127–30.

15. Twickler DM, Riechel T, Mcintire DD, et al. Fetal central nervous system ventricle and cisterna magna measurements by magnetic resonance imaging. Am J Obstet Gynecol 2002;187:927–31.

16. Garel C, Alberti C. Coronal measurement of the fetal lateral ventricles: comparison between ultrasonography and magnetic resonance imaging. Ultrasound Obstet Gynecol 2006;27:23–7.

17. Jou HJ, Shyu MK, Wu SC, et al. Ultrasound measurement of the fetal cavum septi pellucidi. Ultrasound Obstet Gynecol 1998;12:419–21.

18. Falco P, Gabriella S, Visentin A, et al. Transabdominal sonography of the cavum septum pellucidum in normal fetuses in the second and third trimesters of pregnancy. Ultrasound Obstet Gynecol 2000;16:549–53.

19. Sari A, Ahmetoglu A, Dinc H, et al. Fetal biometry: size and configuration of the third ventricle. Acta Radiol 2005;46(6):631–5.

20. Garel C. Fetal cerebral biometry: normal parenchymal findings and ventricular size. Eur Radiol 2005;15:809–13.

21. Goldstein I, Makhoul IR, Tamir A, et al. Ultrasonographic normograms of the fetal fourth ventricle: additional tool for detecting abnormalities of the posterior fossa. J Ultrasound Med 2002;21:849–56.

22. Kinoshita Y, Okudera T, Tsuru E, et al. Volumetric analysis of the germinal matrix and lateral ventricles performed using MR images of postmortem fetuses. AJNR Am J Neuroradiol 2001;22:382–8.

23. Judas M, Rados M, Jovanov-Milosevic N, et al. Structural, immunocytochemical and MR imaging properties of periventricular crossroads of growing cortical pathways in preterm infants. AJNR Am J Neuroradiol 2005;26:2671–784.

24. Pugash D, Hendson G, Dunham CP, et al. Sonographic assessment of normal and abnormal patterns of fetal cerebral lamination. Ultrasound Obstet Gynecol 2012;40:642–51.

25. Brisse H, Fallet C, Sebag G, et al. Supratentorial parenchyma in the developing fetal brain: in vitro MR study with histologic comparison. AJNR Am J Neuroradiol 1997;18:1491–7.

26. Rados M, Judas M, Kostovic I. In vitro MRI of brain development. Eur J Radiol 2006;57:187–98.

27. Widjaja E, Geiprasert S, Mahmoodabadi SZ, et al. Alteration of human fetal subplate layer and intermediate zone during normal development on MR and diffusion tensor imaging. AJNR Am J Neuroradiol 2010;31:1091–9.

28. Levine D, Barnes PD. Cortical maturation in normal and abnormal fetuses as assessed with prenatal MR imaging. Radiology 1999;210:751–8.

29. Monteagudo A, Timor-Tritsch IE. Development of fetal gyri, sulci and fissures: a transvaginal sonographic study. Ultrasound Obstet Gynecol 1997;9:222–8.

30. Kasprian G, Langs G, Brugger PC, et al. The prenatal origin of hemispheric asymmetry: an in utero neuroimaging study. Cereb Cortex 2011;21:1076–83.

31. Pistorius LR, Stoutenbeek P, Groenendaal F, et al. Grade and symmetry of normal fetal cortical development: a longitudinal two and three dimensional ultrasound. Ultrasound Obstet Gynecol 2010;36:700–8.

32. Cohen-Sacher B, Lerman-Sagie T, Lev D, et al. Sonographic developmental milestones of the fetal cortex: a longitudinal study. Ultrasound Obstet Gynecol 2006;27:494–502.

33. Garel C, Chantrel E, Elmaleh M, et al. Fetal MRI: normal gestational landmarks for cerebral biometry, gyration and myelination. Childs Nerv Syst 2003;19:422–5.

34. Youssef A, Ghi T, Pilu G. How to image the fetal corpus callosum. Ultrasound Obstet Gynecol 2014;42(6):718–20.

35. Pashaj S, Merz E, Wellek S. Biometry of the fetal corpus callosum by three-dimensional ultrasound. Ultrasound Obstet Gynecol 2013;42:691–8.

36. Pati M, Cani C, Bertucci E, et al. Early visualization and measurements of the pericallosual artery: an indirect sign of corpus callosum development. J Ultrasound Med 2012;31:231–7.

37. Song JW, Gruber GM, Patsch JM, et al. How accurate are prenatal tractography results? A postnatal in vivo follow-up study using diffusion tensor imaging. Pediatr Radiol 2018;48:486–98.

38. Adamsbaum C, Moutard ML, Andre C, et al. MRI of the fetal posterior fossa. Pediatr Radiol 2005;35:124–40.

39. Mirlesse V, Courtiol C, Althuse M, et al. Untrasonography of the fetal brainstem: a biometric and anatomical, multioperator, cross-sectional study of 913 fetuses of 21-36 weeks of gestation. Prenat Diagn 2010;30:739–45.

40. Bromley B, Nadel AS, Pauker S, et al. Closure of the cerebellar vermis with second trimester US. Radiology 1994;(3):761–3.

41. Volpe P, Contro E, DeMusso F, et al. Brainstem-vermis and brainstem-tentorium angles allow accurate

categorization of fetal upward rotation of cerebellar vermis. Ultrasound Obstet Gynecol 2012;39:632–5.

42. Stazzone MM, Hubbard AM, Bilaniuk LT, et al. Ultrafast MR imaging of the normal posterior fossa in fetuses. AJR Am J Roentgenol 2000; 175:835–9.

43. Robinson AJ, Goldstein R. The cisterna magna septa: vestigial remnants of Blake's pouch and a potential new marker for normal development of the rhombencephalon. J Ultrasound Med 2007;26: 83–95.

44. Triulzi F, Parazzini C, Righini A. MRI of fetal and neonatal cerebellar development. Semin Fetal Neonatal Med 2005;10:411–20.

45. Zalel Y, Yagel S, Achiron R, et al. Three-dimensional ultrasonography of the fetal vermis at 18-26 weeks' gestation. J Ultrasound Med 2009; 28:1–28.

46. Robinson AJ, Blaser S, Toi A, et al. The fetal cerebellar vermis: assessment for abnormal development by ultrasonography and magnetic resonance imaging. Ultrasound Q 2007;23:211–23.

Spinal Dysraphia, Chiari 2 Malformation, Unified Theory, and Advances in Fetoscopic Repair

Jena L. Miller, MD[a],*, Thierry A.G.M. Huisman, MD[b]

KEYWORDS

- Chiari II malformation • Fetoscopy • Fetal surgery • Spina bifida • Prenatal diagnosis

KEY POINTS

- Fetal spina bifida results in lifelong sequelae resulting from both local nerve damage of the exposed spinal cord and treatment of hydrocephalus.
- Prenatal diagnosis reliably made using ultrasonography fetal MR imaging complements the assessment.
- Fetal surgery for spina bifida decreases the need for postnatal ventriculoperintoneal shunt placement and improves motor function.
- Fetoscopic surgery minimizes maternal risks with similar short-term outcomes as open fetal surgery.

INTRODUCTION/SCOPE OF THE CONDITION

Fetal spina bifida is the most common nonlethal birth defect of the central nervous system (CNS) that results when the spinal column and/or neural tube fail to close by the fourth week of gestation.[1] It occurs in about 3 to 4/10,000 live births in the United States and results in significant morbidity and shortened life expectancy.[2] This is predominantly as a result of complications related to sensorineural deficits from the lesion itself and from the short-term and long-term sequelae of an associated hydrocephalus. Prenatal diagnosis of this condition is reliably made using ultrasonography by the second trimester of pregnancy.

UNIFIED THEORY: RELATIONSHIP BETWEEN MYELOMENINGOCELE AND CHIARI 2 MALFORMATION

Fetal spina bifida should be differentiated into 2 major groups; the skin- and nonskin-covered forms. The open, nonskin-covered spina bifida is characterized by a neural placode, which may be in level with the adjacent skin (myelocele) or may be protruding outside of the open spinal canal (myelomeningcele). The neural placode is consequently exposed to the amniotic fluid during pregnancy. The exposure of the neural placode to the amniotic fluid may result in "chemical damage" of the neuronal tissue as well as direct mechanical injury during pregnancy and delivery.[3,4] This complex injury significantly impacts the functionality of the neural placode. In addition, an open neural tube defect is typically linked with a Chiari 2 malformation. The so-called unified theory has recognized the leakage of cerebrospinal fluid out of the open neural tube at the level of the spinal dysraphia into the amniotic fluid as a key etiologic factor for the delayed or ineffective expansion of the rhombencephalic vesicle. Consequently the osseous posterior fossa is too small for its contents, which constitutes the hallmark of a Chiari

Disclosure Statement: The authors have nothing to disclose.
[a] Department of Gynecology and Obstetrics, Johns Hopkins University, 600 North Wolfe Street, Nelson 228, Baltimore, MD 21287, USA; [b] Edward B. Singleton Department of Radiology, Texas Children's Hospital, 6701 Fannin Street, Suite 470, Houston, TX 77030, USA
* Corresponding author.
E-mail address: jmill260@jhmi.edu

2 malformation.[5] On prenatal ultrasonography the Chiari 2 malformation can easily be detected by the lemon-shaped skull configuration as well as the banana-shaped cerebellum on axial imaging.[6,7] High-resolution ultrasonography will usually also depict the tonsillar herniation into the upper spinal canal as well as associated findings including supratentorial hydrocephalus. Fetal MR imaging is complementary to ultrasonography to recognize additional associated findings such as migrational abnormalities or callosal anomalies.[8] The additional findings may significantly impact functional and neurocognitive prognosis. Fetal MR imaging has advanced our understanding of this complex multilevel malformation, which should possibly be reclassified as a fetal disruption rather than a malformation. Further investigations are, however, necessary because the unified theory may explain the combination of the spinal dysraphia and the Chiari 2 malformation, but does not explain the increased incidence of additional cerebral findings such as migrational abnormalities or callosal malformations. Advanced fetal MR imaging including diffusion tensor imaging with tractography may shed more light on this intriguing fetal abnormality.

PRENATAL DIAGNOSIS
First Trimester Ultrasonography

First trimester fetal ultrasonography assessment has tremendous capability for identifying many structural anomalies, including spina bifida, that far surpasses the narrow indication for screening for trisomy 21.[12] Evaluation of the posterior brain can be performed in the same midsagittal plane of the fetal profile that is used to measure the nuchal translucency. Normally, the structures visible in the posterior brain include the brainstem, the fourth ventricle, and the cisterna magna. Several observations, including compression of the fourth ventricle, labeled intracranial translucency, obliteration of cisterna magna, or increase in brain stem to brain stem occipital bone distance, can be used for screening for spina bifida without adding additional time to the first trimester assessment (**Fig. 1**).[13–15] Although the ideal marker for screening for open spina bifida in the first trimester is undefined, prospective evaluation of the posterior brain is feasible and most fetuses will demonstrate some abnormality in this region. Identification of an abnormal appearance in this area can alert the sonographer or clinician that further investigation of the fetal CNS is indicated. Earlier diagnosis maximizes the opportunity for parents to gain sufficient information for management planning, which may include

pregnancy termination, expectant, or fetal surgery.[16]

Maternal Serum Screening

Standard maternal serum screening for fetal spina bifida involves testing for α-fetoprotein, which is secreted from the open spinal dysraphism and crosses the placenta in combination with second trimester ultrasonography anatomic survey. The result of the maternal serum α-fetoprotein is expressed as a multiple of the median (MoM) corrected for maternal ethnicity, fetal number, maternal weight, and presence of diabetes. The MoM is then translated into the a priori risk for the specific pregnancy.[9] Increased maternal serum α-fetoprotein can occur with other fetal anomalies, such as abdominal wall defects, the detection rate is anticipated to be greater than 95% and up to 80% for open spina bifida, with a false-positive rate of 1% to 3% when a threshold of 2.5 MoM is used.[10] Knowledge of this test result before second trimester ultrasonography may increase the level of scrutiny that must be applied to evaluating the fetal CNS during the examination; however, it is not a requisite that substantially improves detection on prenatal ultrasonography.[11]

Second Trimester Ultrasonography

Second trimester ultrasonography is the diagnostic test for fetal spina bifida and can identify up to 96% of cases. Classic ultrasonography findings of the fetal head include bitemporal narrowing of the frontal bones (lemon sign),

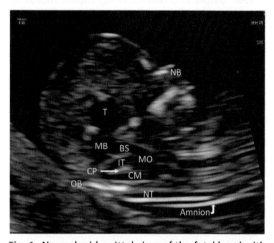

Fig. 1. Normal midsagittal view of the fetal head with major landmarks identified. The amnion is identified by the arrow. BS, brainstem; CM, cisterna magna; CP, choroid plexus; IT, intracranial translucency; MB, midbrain; MO, medulla oblongata; NB, nasal bone; NT, nuchal translucency; OB, occipital bone; T, thalamus.

semicircular shape of the cerebellum with or without obliteration of the posterior fossa (banana sign), and possibly ventriculomegaly (**Fig. 2**).[6,7] The biparietal diameter and head circumference may be small or large for gestational age based on the presence of ventriculomegaly. The spine must be assessed in both the sagittal and transverse planes to evaluate for abnormalities[17–19] (**Fig. 3**). The most common location for spina bifida is within the lumbosacral region, but small or flat lesions can be challenging to detect at any level.

Level Localization

Once the defect is identified, determining the upper border of the bony lesion, and whether or not it is skin covered, and if kyphosis is present, are the most important factors for family counseling.[20] Presence or absence of additional anomalies are important features to consider to verify if the spina bifida is isolated or potentially part of a more complex fetal condition such as aneuploidy or genetic syndrome.[21,22]

The addition of 3-dimensional ultrasonography may help to delineate the appearance of the lesion and relationship between the level of the bone and skin defect (**Fig. 4**). Optimal image acquisition involves capturing the fetus in a dorsoanterior position during complete quiescence with an amniotic fluid interface over the region of interest. The sweep is acquired using a sagittal plane with narrow angle and maximum quality.[23] The volume can then be manipulated in the render and multiplanar modes either off-line or on the machine. In the multiplanar mode, the image is rotated so that the coronal, sagittal, and transverse views are optimally visualized in each window. On the skeletal mode (mix 10/90 of surface/max) the 12th rib is identified on the coronal image and the reference point can be moved gradually along the spine at each vertebral level until the level of bony splaying is seen on the transverse view. Similarly, the skin defect can be identified by activating the soft tissue preset (mix 30/70 or 50/50 of surface/max), and the skin level can be marked and measured in the sagittal image.[24] Compared with 2-dimensional ultrasonography assessment, use of multiplanar

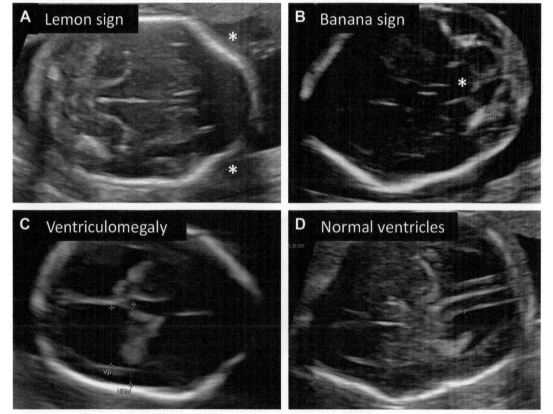

Fig. 2. Secondary intracranial signs of fetal spina bifida. (*A*) Bitemporal narrowing of the frontal bones resembling the shape of a lemon (*asterisks*). (*B*) The concave appearance of the cerebellum is referred to as the banana sign (*asterisk*). (*C*) Either ventriculomegaly (>10 mm) or (*D*) normal ventricle size may be observed with fetal spina bifida.

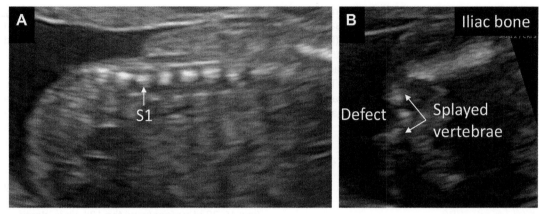

Fig. 3. Fetal myeloschisis with upper border at S1 (*arrows*) visualized in both the sagittal (*A*) and transverse (*B*) planes.

evaluation of the upper border of the lesion is complementary and shows good agreement to postnatal imaging within 1 vertebral level in nearly all prospectively evaluated fetuses.[23,25]

Functional Assessment

Progressive loss of neurologic function and development of talipes is a common observation during pregnancy.[4,26] Attention to mobility of the hips, knees, and ankles, and foot position, during the ultrasonography assessment provides a surrogate marker for the level of preserved neurologic function on the postnatal examination. This technique showed good agreement for both the right and left lower extremities of 91.7% and 88.9% for the right and left lower extremities, respectively (Fig. 5).[27] In addition, the technique shows a high level of agreement between observers of various levels of expertise after only a short training period.[28] Other markers used for patient

counseling regarding the potential for ambulation include muscle wasting in the lower extremities and position of the extremities (Fig. 6).[20]

Ultrasonography remains the primary diagnostic and assessment modality to determine treatment eligibility, but fetal MR imaging is a critical adjunct to evaluate specific characteristics of the anomaly, verify hindbrain herniation, and assess for additional brain malformations or migrational disorders that impact prognosis. The pertinent positive and negative findings on fetal MR imaging that are critical for counseling, pregnancy management, and longitudinal assessment are described in Table 1.

FETAL MR IMAGING FOR SPINA BIFIDA

Typically, a triplanar (axial, coronal, and sagittal to the mother) "scout" sequence (eg, TRUE fast imaging with steady-state precession sequence) is acquired at the beginning of the MR imaging study. These sequences allow to position the

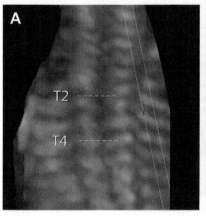
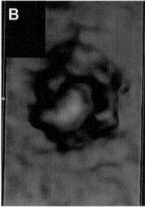
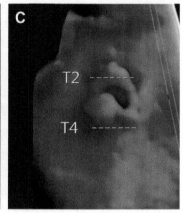

Fig. 4. Three-dimensional ultrasonography volume with surface rendering of a thoracic myelocele. The level of the lesion is annotated on the coronal plane in the skeletal mode (*A*). Surface rendering (*B*) or high-definition live mode (*C*) is activated revealing the contour of the lesion.

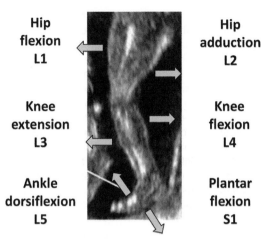

Hip flexion L1 — Hip adduction L2

Knee extension L3 — Knee flexion L4

Ankle dorsiflexion L5 — Plantar flexion S1

Fig. 5. Segmental evaluation of lower extremity motor function. Observation of fetal lower extremity movement in real-time provides a functional assessment of the lesion from L1 to S1.

subsequent high-resolution sequences adapted to the position of the fetus. In addition, these fast, nonbreath-hold sequences give valuable preliminary anatomic information about the fetus and its position. These scout sequences are followed by high-resolution, dedicated T2-weighted ultrafast single-shot fast spin echo or half Fourier single-shot turbo spin echo sequences similar to the well reported T2-weighted sequences typically used for fetal brain anatomy. The single-slice acquisition and ultrafast acquisition times (≤500 ms per slice) allow to "picture freeze" the intrauterine fetus. The T2-weighted sequences have an excellent contrast-to-noise and signal-to-noise ratio. The fetal CNS and spinal cord are still very "watery," resulting in a strong MR imaging signal. In addition, the spinal cord and canal is well depicted because the spinal cord is outlined by the T2-hyperintense cerebrospinal fluid. Multiplanar imaging is necessary to study the exact anatomy of the normal and abnormal spinal cord. Focal lesions may go undetected if only 1 imaging plane is measured.

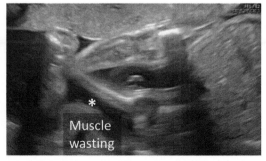

*

Muscle wasting

Fig. 6. Bilateral clubbed feet with evidence of muscle wasting in the inferior lower leg (*asterisk*).

Table 1
Pertinent positive and negative findings for spina bifida ideally reported on MR imaging

	Positive	Negative
Fetal brain	Ventriculomegaly[a] Presence of corpus callosum Chiari malformation/ grade[a] Obliteration of cisterna magna[a] Visibility of 4th ventricle[a]	Additional abnormalities Heterotopia
Fetal spine/ extremities	Open vs closed lesion[a] Upper level of defect Dimensions	Kyphosis Syrinx Epidermoid cyst[b]
Maternal structures	Uterine anomaly	

[a] Preoperative and 6-week postoperative examination.
[b] Postnatal.

T1-weighted imaging is limited because currently no ultrafast single-shot T1-weighted sequences are available. T1-weighted imaging may, however, be essential to identify T1-hyperintense fat, as seen in cases of a lipomeningomyelocele or intradural lipomas.

Dynamic T2-weighted sequences may be added to the standard anatomic sequences to get a global overview of the motion of, for example, the lower extremities in fetuses with a spinal dysraphia. It is, however, well known that active "moonwalking" (in honor of Michael Jackson) does not correlate well with final functional outcome.

It is a sine qua non that the entire CNS should always be evaluated. A nonskin-covered spinal dysraphia is nearly always associated with an Arnold-Chiari 2 malformation. Occasionally the spinal dysraphia may be difficult to recognize, in this scenario identification of an Arnold-Chiari 2 malformation may indicate a coexisting spinal dysraphia. Finally, in spinal dysraphia not only should the entire CNS be carefully studied but also the remainder of the fetal anatomy to rule out associated orthopedic, gastrointestinal, or genitourinary anomalies.

PREGNANCY MANAGEMENT AND FETAL SURGERY

Once any fetal anomaly such as spina bifida is identified, the pregnancy is considered high-risk because alterations of maternal or fetal care may be required for the specific condition. The care path of a pregnancy complicated with fetal spina bifida involves consultation with a maternal fetal medicine specialist, genetic counseling, and consideration of diagnostic testing with amniocentesis or chorionic villus sampling, depending on gestational age.

Historically, postnatal surgery was performed to close the defect within the first 2 days of birth. The randomized Management of Myelomeningocele Study (MOMS) sparked a paradigm shift establishing that prenatal surgery was beneficial to decrease the rate of ventriculomegaly and subsequent ventriculoperitoneal shunting by 1 year (82%–40%) of age and improved rate of independent ambulation (21%–42%) for selected fetuses.[29]

Inclusion criteria for prenatal surgery included fetuses with:

- Isolated spina bifida (upper border T1-S1)
- 19 + 6 to 25 + 6 weeks gestation
- Evidence of hindbrain herniation
- Normal karyotype

Although fetal benefit was demonstrated, these children experienced a higher preterm birth rate (34 + 1 weeks vs 37 + 3 weeks), higher incidence of respiratory distress, and lower birth weight. Maternal obstetric and surgical risks associated with the procedure are respectable and include mandatory cesarean delivery, pulmonary edema, placental abruption, blood transfusion at delivery, and the potential for scar complications including rupture and dehiscence of up to 14% at the hysterotomy site for the index and every future pregnancy.[29–32]

INFRASTRUCTURE FOR PRENATAL SURGERY

Only 3 experienced centers in open maternal and fetal surgery participated in the MOMS trial. During this time all other fetal therapy centers in the United States agreed to halt performing this procedure until the trial was complete. Once the benefit of prenatal surgery for spina bifida was established, demand and availability of the technique rapidly expanded. To provide the framework for centers to offer prenatal repair safely and establish the standard of care that centers should uphold, the MMC (myelomeningocele) Task Force was created with representatives from the professional organizations of all aspects of maternal, fetal, and pediatric care for fetal spina bifida.[33] These guidelines require that a fetal team be comprised of members with adequate expertise in their respective fields to provide appropriate interdisciplinary assessment, counseling, surgical planning, pregnancy management, and postnatal follow-up (Box 1). Importantly, the team must have an established working relationship and receive adequate training or guidance from an experienced center before implementation of a prenatal spina bifida repair program that adheres to the MOMS trial inclusion and exclusion criteria. Because spina bifida is a lifelong chronic condition, the center must be associated with or able to provide long-term care through a designated spina bifida clinic. To determine if results from the MOMS trial are generalizable to clinical practice and that outcomes are durable, participation in a national registry and ongoing quality assessment is necessary.

TECHNIQUES FOR PRENATAL REPAIR

Fetal surgery for spina bifida is performed within the second trimester of pregnancy. This balances the lower risk for preterm labor and aims to prevent ongoing nerve damage during the remainder of the pregnancy. The optimal time to minimize the risk for chorion amnion separation or premature rupture of membranes seems to be beyond 23 weeks.[34] The surgical approach falls into 2 major categories, either through open fetal surgery,[35] or by fetoscopy, which is minimally invasive to the uterus.[36–42] Early attempts using fetoscopy were largely abandoned because of suboptimal outcomes,[43] but there has been a resurgence of interest in fetoscopy due to the significant short-term and long-term maternal risks of open fetal surgery.

Open fetal surgery is performed under general anesthesia through a laparotomy on the maternal abdomen followed by exteriorization of the uterus. Fetal and placental location are verified by ultrasonography performed directly on the uterus to

---

Box 1
Multispecialty team requirements for prenatal spina bifida repair

- Maternal Fetal Medicine with advanced ultrasonography expertise
- Pediatric Radiology with fetal MR imaging capability and expertise
- Fetal echocardiography
- Fetal surgeon—either Maternal Fetal Medicine or Pediatric Surgery
- Pediatric Neurosurgery
- Obstetric/Pediatric Anesthesiology
- Neonatology
- Fetal care coordinator
- Social work

determine the optimal location for the hysterotomy. Next, full-thickness sutures are placed through the uterus and membranes with ultrasound guidance and a small opening is created using cautery. The uterine incision is extended on each side using absorbable staples so that a hemostatic opening is created that is large enough to expose the fetal back. The fetal back is elevated to the incision and then the repair is performed directly on the lesion. Fetal heart rate and cardiac function is monitored continuously by ultrasonography through the uterus. Once completed, the fetus is lowered back into the uterus, adequate amniotic fluid volume is verified, and the uterus is closed in layers. The maternal abdomen is closed using standard technique.[35]

In contrast, the fetoscopic approach uses between 2 and 4 ports introduced directly into the uterus with ultrasound guidance either percutaneously or via maternal laparotomy. Amnioreduction followed by partial carbon dioxide insufflation is used to provide a dry working environment for the repair.[44] Initial reports using a completely percutaneous approach demonstrated that the

technique was feasible but had longer operative times, a higher rate of premature rupture of membranes and preterm birth compared with open fetal surgery.[36,37,40] Alternatively, open fetoscopy is a hybrid technique that involves port placement in the exteriorized uterus. This allows fixation of the membranes to the uterine wall thereby contributing to a more acceptable rate of ruptured membranes[41,42,45] and alleviates the difference in prematurity compared with open fetal surgery in a recent meta-analysis (Fig. 7).[46] No uterine scar complications have been reported in any of the fetoscopic series, allowing labor management and mode of delivery to be determined by standard obstetric indications.[47]

The fetoscopic approach is obstetrically safer for the mother but to be considered equivalent to standard open fetal surgery similar neurologic outcomes must be demonstrated. Achieving a watertight closure of the defect seems to be the most important factor for improving cerebrospinal fluid dynamics and reversing hindbrain herniation.[48,49] The open fetal surgical technique aims to replicate the steps of postnatal closure,[35] however the

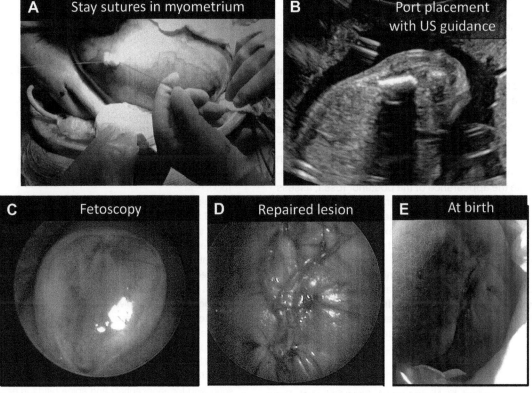

Fig. 7. Two port open fetoscopy performed via maternal laparotomy and exteriorized uterus. Ports are secured with stay sutures through the myometrium (*A*) using ultrasound guidance (*B*). The lesion is visualized using fetoscopy (*C*) and repaired with a series of interrupted sutures (*D*). Typical appearance of the surgical site after vaginal delivery at term (*E*).

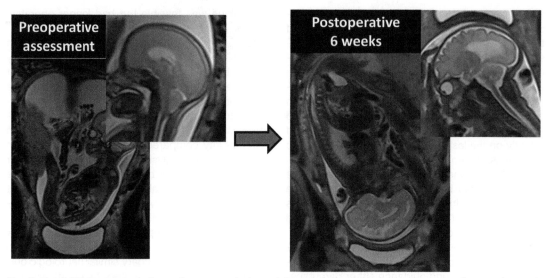

Fig. 8. Fetal MR imaging performed preoperatively and 6 weeks postoperatively after open fetoscopic repair. Midsagittal view demonstrates obliteration of the cisterna magna, downward displacement of the cerebellum, and effacement of the fourth ventricle. Interval improvement in hindbrain herniation and restoration of the CSF-filled spaces observed. CSF, cerebrospinal fluid.

various fetoscopic techniques achieve closure using either fewer layers or incorporate additional barrier materials in attempt to minimize cord tethering at the repair site.[38–42,45,50] Short-term outcomes are similar between fetoscopic and open techniques with greater than 70% of fetuses showing improvement of hindbrain herniation[32,40] (Fig. 8) and reduction of ventriculoperitoneal shunt rate of 43% to 45% after fetoscopy[40,51] compared with 40% in the MOMS trial.[29] Long-term follow-up of these children is required to determine if similar gains in motor function are achieved as well as the need for postnatal revision or reoperation. Follow-up MR imaging can be performed in the newborn period and during childhood to evaluate the appearance of the posterior fossa, assess for additional brain or migrational abnormalities that may have been suspected prenatally and complement the physical examination if there is concern for clinical cord tethering, epidermoid cyst, or syrinx formation.[52–54] An international consortium of centers performing fetoscopic spina bifida repair has been created to foster shared experience and provide the framework for streamlining data collection and evaluating the longer-term effects of this technique.[55]

REFERENCES

1. Wallingford JB, Niswander LA, Shaw GM, et al. The continuing challenge of understanding, preventing, and treating neural tube defects. Science 2013; 339(6123):1222002.

2. Williams J, Mai CT, Mulinare JT, et al. Updated estimates of neural tube defects prevented by mandatory folic acid fortification — United States, 1995–2011. MMWR Morb Mortal Wkly Rep 2015; 64:1–5.

3. Hutchins GM, Meuli M, Meuli-Simmen C, et al. Acquired spinal cord injury in human fetuses with myelomeningocele. Pediatr Pathol Lab Med 1996;16(5): 701–12.

4. Meuli M, Meuli-Simmen C, Yingling CD, et al. Creation of myelomeningocele in utero: a model of functional damage from spinal cord exposure in fetal sheep. J Pediatr Surg 1995;30(7):1028–33.

5. McLone DG, Knepper PA. The cause of Chiari II malformation: a unified theory. Pediatr Neurosci 1989; 15(1):1–12.

6. Nicolaides KH, Campbell S, Gabbe SG, et al. Ultrasound screening for spina bifida: cranial and cerebellar signs. Lancet 1986;2(8498):72–4.

7. Van den Hof MC, Nicolaides KH, Campbell J, et al. Evaluation of the lemon and banana signs in one hundred thirty fetuses with open spina bifida. Am J Obstet Gynecol 1990;162(2):322–7.

8. Trigubo D, Negri M, Salvatico RM, et al. The role of intrauterine magnetic resonance in the management of myelomenigocele. Childs Nerv Syst 2017;33(7): 1107–11.

9. Wald NJ, Cuckle H, Brock JH, et al. Maternal serum-alpha-fetoprotein measurement in antenatal screening for anencephaly and spina bifida in early pregnancy. Report of U.K. collaborative study on alpha-fetoprotein in relation to neural-tube defects. Lancet 1977;1(8026):1323–32.

10. Bradley LA, Palomaki GE, McDowell GA. Technical standards and guidelines: prenatal screening for open neural tube defects: this new section on "Prenatal Screening for Open Neural Tube Defects," together with the new section on "Prenatal Screening for Down Syndrome," replaces the previous Section H of the American College of Medical Genetics Standards and Guidelines for Clinical Genetics Laboratories*. Genet Med 2005;7:355.

11. Norem CT, Schoen EJ, Walton DL, et al. Routine ultrasonography compared with maternal serum alpha-fetoprotein for neural tube defect screening. Obstet Gynecol 2005;106(4):747–52.

12. Souka AP, Pilalis A, Kavalakis Y, et al. Assessment of fetal anatomy at the 11-14-week ultrasound examination. Ultrasound Obstet Gynecol 2004;24(7):730–4.

13. Chaoui R, Benoit B, Mitkowska-Wozniak H, et al. Assessment of intracranial translucency (IT) in the detection of spina bifida at the 11-13-week scan. Ultrasound Obstet Gynecol 2009;34(3):249–52.

14. Lachmann R, Chaoui R, Moratalla J, et al. Posterior brain in fetuses with open spina bifida at 11 to 13 weeks. Prenat Diagn 2011;31(1):103–6.

15. Papastefanou I, Souka AP, Pilalis A, et al. Fetal intracranial translucency and cisterna magna at 11 to 14 weeks: reference ranges and correlation with chromosomal abnormalities. Prenat Diagn 2011;31(12):1189–92.

16. Orlandi E, Rossi C, Perino A, et al. Prospective sonographic detection of spina bifida at 11-14 weeks and systematic literature review. J Matern Fetal Neonatal Med 2016;29(14):2363–7.

17. American Institute of Ultrasound in Medicine. AIUM practice guideline for the performance of obstetric ultrasound examinations. J Ultrasound Med 2013;32(6):1083–101.

18. Salomon LJ, Alfirevic Z, Berghella V, et al. Practice guidelines for performance of the routine mid-trimester fetal ultrasound scan. Ultrasound Obstet Gynecol 2011;37(1):116–26.

19. International Society of Ultrasound in Obstetrics & Gynecology Education Committee. Sonographic examination of the fetal central nervous system: guidelines for performing the "basic examination" and the "fetal neurosonogram." Ultrasound Obstet Gynecol 2007;29(1):109–16.

20. Coleman BG, Langer JE, Horii SC. The diagnostic features of spina bifida: the role of ultrasound. Fetal Diagn Ther 2015;37(3):179–96.

21. Mitchell LE, Adzick NS, Melchionne J, et al. Spina bifida. Lancet 2004;364(9448):1885–95.

22. Sepulveda W, Corral E, Ayala C, et al. Chromosomal abnormalities in fetuses with open neural tube defects: prenatal identification with ultrasound. Ultrasound Obstet Gynecol 2004;23(4):352–6.

23. Buyukkurt S, Binokay F, Seydaoglu G, et al. Prenatal determination of the upper lesion level of spina bifida with three-dimensional ultrasound. Fetal Diagn Ther 2013;33(1):36–40.

24. Faden MS, Miller JL, Baschat AA. Annotation-assisted multiplanar volume contrast imaging (VCI) to assess the level of fetal meningomyelocele: electronic poster abstracts. Ultrasound Obstet Gynecol 2018;52:224.

25. Lee W, Chaiworapongsa T, Romero R, et al. A diagnostic approach for the evaluation of spina bifida by three-dimensional ultrasonography. J Ultrasound Med 2002;21(6):619–26.

26. Stiefel D, Copp AJ, Meuli M. Fetal spina bifida in a mouse model: loss of neural function in utero. J Neurosurg 2007;106(3 Suppl):213–21.

27. Carreras E, Maroto A, Illescas T, et al. Prenatal ultrasound evaluation of segmental level of neurological lesion in fetuses with myelomeningocele: development of a new technique. Ultrasound Obstet Gynecol 2016;47(2):162–7.

28. Maroto A, Illescas T, Meléndez M, et al. Ultrasound functional evaluation of fetuses with myelomeningocele: study of the interpretation of results. J Matern Fetal Neonatal Med 2017;30(19):2301–5.

29. Adzick NS, Thom EA, Spong CY, et al. A randomized trial of prenatal versus postnatal repair of myelomeningocele. N Engl J Med 2011;364(11):993–1004.

30. Wilson RD, Lemerand K, Johnson MP, et al. Reproductive outcomes in subsequent pregnancies after a pregnancy complicated by open maternal-fetal surgery (1996-2007). Am J Obstet Gynecol 2010;203(3):209.e1-6.

31. Johnson MP, Bennett KA, Rand L, et al. The Management of Myelomeningocele Study: obstetrical outcomes and risk factors for obstetrical complications following prenatal surgery. Am J Obstet Gynecol 2016;215(6):778.e1-9.

32. Moldenhauer JS, Soni S, Rintoul NE, et al. Fetal myelomeningocele repair: the post-MOMS experience at the Children's Hospital of Philadelphia. Fetal Diagn Ther 2015;37(3):235–40.

33. Cohen AR, Couto J, Cummings JJ, et al. Position statement on fetal myelomeningocele repair. Am J Obstet Gynecol 2014;210(2):107–11.

34. Wilson RD, Johnson MP, Crombleholme TM, et al. Chorioamniotic membrane separation following open fetal surgery: pregnancy outcome. Fetal Diagn Ther 2003;18(5):314–20.

35. Heuer GG, Adzick NS, Sutton LN. Fetal myelomeningocele closure: technical considerations. Fetal Diagn Ther 2015;37(3):166–71.

36. Kohl T, Hering R, Heep A, et al. Percutaneous fetoscopic patch coverage of spina bifida aperta in the human–early clinical experience and potential. Fetal Diagn Ther 2006;21(2):185–93.

37. Verbeek RJ, Heep A, Maurits NM, et al. Fetal endoscopic myelomeningocele closure preserves segmental neurological function. Dev Med Child Neurol 2012;54(1):15–22.

38. Kohl T. Percutaneous minimally invasive fetoscopic surgery for spina bifida aperta. Part I: surgical technique and perioperative outcome. Ultrasound Obstet Gynecol 2014;44(5):515–24.

39. Pedreira DAL, Zanon N, Nishikuni K, et al. Endoscopic surgery for the antenatal treatment of myelomeningocele: the CECAM trial. Am J Obstet Gynecol 2016;214(1):111.e1-11.

40. Lapa Pedreira DA, Acacio GL, Gonçalves RT, et al. Percutaneous fetoscopic closure of large open spina bifida using a bilaminar skin substitute. Ultrasound Obstet Gynecol 2018. https://doi.org/10.1002/uog.19001.

41. Belfort MA, Whitehead WE, Shamshirsaz AA, et al. Fetoscopic open neural tube defect repair: development and refinement of a two-port, carbon dioxide insufflation technique. Obstet Gynecol 2017;129(4):734–43.

42. Giné C, Arévalo S, Maíz N, et al. Fetoscopic two-layers closure of open neural tube defects. Ultrasound Obstet Gynecol 2018. https://doi.org/10.1002/uog.19104.

43. Bruner JP, Richards WO, Tulipan NB, et al. Endoscopic coverage of fetal myelomeningocele in utero. Am J Obstet Gynecol 1999;180(1 Pt 1):153–8.

44. Kohl T, Tchatcheva K, Weinbach J, et al. Partial amniotic carbon dioxide insufflation (PACI) during minimally invasive fetoscopic surgery: early clinical experience in humans. Surg Endosc 2010;24(2):432–44.

45. Miller JL, Groves M, Faden M, et al. Performance of open two-port fetoscopic fetal spina bifida repair in a newly developed program. Am J Obstet Gynecol 2019;S1:S149–50.

46. Kabagambe SK, Jensen GW, Chen YJ, et al. Fetal surgery for myelomeningocele: a systematic review and meta-analysis of outcomes in fetoscopic versus open repair. Fetal Diagn Ther 2018;43(3):161–74.

47. Kohn JR, Rao V, Sellner AA, et al. Management of labor and delivery after fetoscopic repair of an open neural tube defect. Obstet Gynecol 2018;131(6):1062–8.

48. Meuli M, Moehrlen U. Fetal surgery for myelomeningocele: a critical appraisal. Eur J Pediatr Surg 2013;23(2):103–9.

49. Peranteau WH, Adzick NS. Prenatal surgery for myelomeningocele. Curr Opin Obstet Gynecol 2016;28(2):111–8.

50. Herrera SRF, Leme RJ, Valente PR, et al. Comparison between two surgical techniques for prenatal correction of meningomyelocele in sheep. Einstein (Sao Paulo) 2012;10(4):455–61.

51. Graf K, Kohl T, Neubauer BA, et al. Percutaneous minimally invasive fetoscopic surgery for spina bifida aperta. Part III: neurosurgical intervention in the first postnatal year. Ultrasound Obstet Gynecol 2016;47(2):158–61.

52. Heye P, Moehrlen U, Mazzone L, et al. Inclusion cysts after fetal spina bifida repair: a third hit? Fetal Diagn Ther 2018. https://doi.org/10.1159/000491877.

53. Bixenmann BJ, Kline-Fath BM, Bierbrauer KS, et al. Prenatal and postnatal evaluation for syringomyelia in patients with spinal dysraphism. J Neurosurg Pediatr 2014;14(3):316–21.

54. Danzer E, Adzick NS, Rintoul NE, et al. Intradural inclusion cysts following in utero closure of myelomeningocele: clinical implications and follow-up findings. J Neurosurg Pediatr 2008;2(6):406–13.

55. Miller JL, Groves ML, Baschat AA. Fetoscopic spina bifida repair. Minerva Ginecol 2018. https://doi.org/10.23736/S0026-4784.18.04355-1.

Posterior Fossa Malformations

Mariasavina Severino, MD[a],*, Thierry A.G.M. Huisman, MD[b]

KEYWORDS

- Brain stem • Cerebellum • Midbrain-hindbrain • Malformations • Neuroimaging • MR imaging • DTI
- Children

KEY POINTS

- Progress in neuroimaging and genetics in the last decades has led to a significant improvement/refinement in the definition/classification of cerebellar and brainstem malformations.
- Neuroimaging plays a key role in the diagnostic workup of children with cerebellar and brainstem malformations.
- Advanced neuroimaging techniques, such as diffusion tensor imaging, have greatly improved the characterization of posterior fossa malformations, demonstrating white matter tract anomalies due to disrupted or altered axonal path-finding.

INTRODUCTION

Posterior fossa malformations include a wide spectrum of heterogeneous conditions caused by disruption of molecular pathways involved in cerebellar and brainstem formation, secondary to gene mutations, teratogens, or combined effects.[1–3] In the last few decades, progress in neuroimaging techniques, neurogenetic analysis, and mouse model research has led to a significant improvement in the definition and classification of these malformations as well as in the recognition of novel disorders. Several classification schemes have been proposed based on neuroimaging, molecular/genetic criteria, and developmental biological criteria.[1–3] However, posterior fossa malformations remain a challenging diagnosis, because they are uncommon and less well known compared with supratentorial anomalies. Moreover, children present with a wide spectrum of neurologic and systemic manifestations, resulting in a highly variable clinical phenotype.[1,2] Therefore, knowledge of neuroimaging features is fundamental for recognizing these malformations correctly.[1–5]

Here, the authors discuss imaging techniques and protocols, describe the normal anatomy of the posterior fossa and its contents, and review the characteristic neuroimaging features of posterior fossa malformations, based on a simplified classification: (a) Predominantly cerebellar malformations, (b) Combined cerebellar and brainstem malformations, and (c) Predominantly brainstem malformations.[2]

IMAGING TECHNIQUES AND NORMAL ANATOMY

MR imaging is the imaging modality of choice allowing detailed evaluation of the anatomy of the posterior fossa and its contents (**Fig. 1A–C, Table 1**).[1–3] Computed tomography has a limited role and is mainly used for the detection of bony anomalies and/or calcifications that may remain undetected on MR imaging. In the last decade, advanced MR imaging techniques, such as diffusion tensor imaging (DTI) and fiber tractography (FT), allowed in vivo demonstration of normal brainstem and cerebellar microstructural anatomy (**Fig. 1D–G**). DTI and FT proved to be especially

Disclosure: The authors have nothing to disclose.
[a] Neuroradiology Unit, IRCCS Istituto Giannina Gaslini, via Gaslini 5, Genoa 16147, Italy; [b] Edward B. Singleton Department of Radiology, Texas Children's Hospital, 6701 Fannin Street, Suite 470, Houston, TX 77030, USA
* Corresponding author.
E-mail address: MariasavinaSeverino@gaslini.org

Neuroimag Clin N Am 29 (2019) 367–383
https://doi.org/10.1016/j.nic.2019.03.008

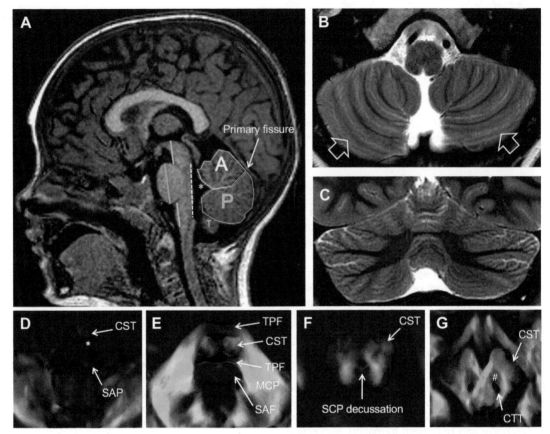

Fig. 1. Normal posterior fossa anatomy. (*A*) On midline sagittal T1-weighted MR imaging, the rostrocaudal length of the ventral pons (*blue line*) is approximately 1.5 that of the midbrain, whereas the rostrocaudal length of the midbrain should be roughly the same as that of the medulla (*orange lines*). The posterior margin of the brainstem extending from the caudal sylvian aqueduct to the obex should be a straight line (*dotted line*). The fastigium should lie just below the midpoint of the ventral pons (*asterisks*). The vermis is divided into anterior (A) and posterior (P) parts by the primary fissure. (*B*) Axial and (*C*) coronal T2-weighted MR images show the normal size and morphology of the cerebellar hemispheres. The cerebellar folia run parallel to the calvarium (onionlike configuration; *arrows*). Coronal images show fissures radiating toward the cerebellar nuclei. (*D–G*) Axial directionally encoded color fractional anisotropy (FA) maps, magnified view at 4 brainstem levels (rostral medulla, middle pons, middle midbrain, and rostral midbrain). Conventional color scheme: blue (inferior-superior), green (anteroposterior), and red (left-right). CCT, central tegmental tract; CST, corticospinal tract; MCP, middle cerebellar peduncles; SAF, somatosensory ascending fibers; TPF, transverse pontocerebellar fibers. *, Inferior olivary nucleus; #, red nucleus.

helpful to study white matter anomalies secondary to axonal path-finding disorders.[4–7] Finally, congenital abnormalities of the cerebellum and brainstem are progressively diagnosed by prenatal ultrasound and MR imaging. Fetal MR imaging generally includes single-shot T2-weighted, T1-weighted, and diffusion-weighted sequences.[8]

Predominantly Cerebellar Malformations

Dandy-Walker malformation

Dandy-Walker malformation (DWM) is defined by a cystic enlargement of the fourth ventricle associated with hypoplasia/agenesis of the vermis. It occurs sporadically in 1:25,000 to 35,000 live births.[9–11] Patients present in the first months of life with symptoms of intracranial hypertension and macrocephaly. DWM may be isolated or may be part of numerous chromosomal anomalies or Mendelian disorders. Interestingly, FOXC1 mutations resulting in dysgenesis of both the cerebellum and its overlying mesenchyme may cause DWM.[9]

On imaging, DWM is characterized by the following[10,11]:

- Upward and counterclockwise rotation of a hypoplastic/agenetic superior vermis
- Cystic dilatation of the fourth ventricle

Table 1
Recommended diagnostic MR imaging protocol

Sequence	Plane	Key Role
Isotropic 3D T1-WI	Multiplanar reformation	High-resolution anatomic information
2 or 3 mm 2D T2-WI	Axial, coronal	Detailed evaluation of cerebellar foliation, cortex, gray-white matter differentiation, dentate and cranial nerve nuclei
2D or 3D FLAIR images	Axial, coronal	Depiction of signal abnormalities
3D heavily T2-WI (CISS, DRIVE, FIESTA)	Multiplanar reformation	Evaluation of cranial nerves, inner ear, ventricular outlets
Susceptibility-weighted imaging	Axial	Highly sensitive for blood products and calcifications
DTI FT	Multiplanar reformation	Qualitative and quantitative information about white matter microstructure and architecture

Abbreviations: CISS, constructive interference in steady state; DRIVE, driven equilibrium; FIESTA, Fast Imaging Employing Steady-state Acquisition; FLAIR, Fluid Attenuated Inversion Recovery; WI, weighted images.

- Enlarged posterior fossa with varying degrees of upward displacement of transverse sinuses, tentorium, and torcular Herophili ("torcular-lambdoid inversion")
- Variable hypoplasia and anterolateral displacement of the cerebellar hemispheres
- Supratentorial hydrocephalus (about 90% of cases)
- Additional brain malformations, including callosal dysgenesis or agenesis, occipital encephalocele, polymicrogyria, and gray matter heterotopias (30%–50% of patients).

The first 3 findings are consistently present and required for diagnosis (**Fig. 2**).

In addition, various anomalies may coexist outside of the central nervous system (CNS), including polydactyly and cardiac anomalies.

Differential diagnoses of DWM include the following (**Fig. 3, Table 2**):

- Blake pouch cyst
- Mega cisterna magna
- Posterior fossa arachnoid cyst
- Isolated vermian hypoplasia

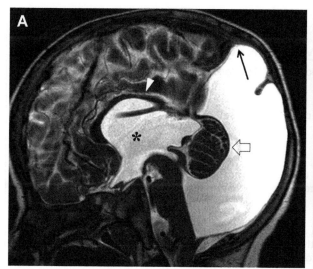
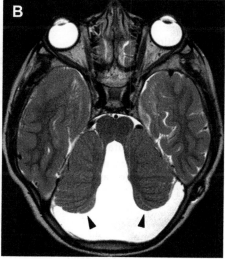

Fig. 2. DWM. (*A*) Sagittal and (*B*) axial T2-weighted MR images show upward and counterclockwise rotation of a hypoplastic vermis (*open arrow*), cystic dilatation of the fourth ventricle, lateral displacement of cerebellar hemispheres (*black arrowheads*), and torcular-lamboid inversion (*arrow*). Note the supratentorial hydrocephalus (*asterisk*), callosal hypoplasia (*white arrowhead*), and hypertelorism.

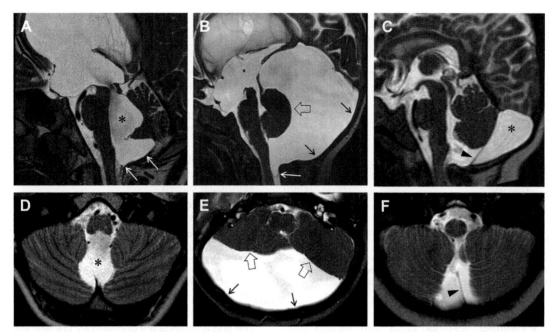

Fig. 3. Posterior fossa cystic malformations. (A) Midsagittal and (D) axial T2-weighted MR images of a child with a Blake pouch cyst reveal enlargement of the fourth ventricle (*asterisks*), which communicates with an infravermian cystic compartment corresponding to the Blake pouch cyst (*arrows*), a normal vermis, and tetraventricular hydrocephalus. (B) Midsagittal and (E) axial T2-weighted MR images of a child with a retrovermian arachnoid cyst demonstrate a CSF isointense cyst with posterior fossa enlargement, occipital bone scalloping (*black arrows*), mass effect on normal-appearing vermis and hemispheres (*open arrows*), normal fourth ventricle, and supratentorial hydrocephalus. Note the inferior cystic wall herniating through the foramen magnum (*white arrow*). (C) Midsagittal and (F) axial T2-weighted MR images of a child with megacisterna magna (*asterisk*) show normal vermis, fourth ventricle, and posterior fossa, remnants of the falx cerebelli (*arrowhead*), and absence of hydrocephalus.

Table 2
Differential diagnosis of cystic posterior fossa malformations

Malformation	Vermis	Fourth Ventricle	Posterior Fossa	Hydrocephalus	Occipital Scalloping
DWM	Hypoplastic, markedly rotated	Enlarged	Enlarged	Frequent	Yes
BPC	Normal, slightly upward rotated	Enlarged	Normal	Frequent	No
MCM	Normal, not rotated	Normal	Normal or slightly enlarged	Absent	Possible
PFAC	Normal (occasionally compressed), not rotated	Normal or reduced	Normal or slightly enlarged	Rare	Yes
IVH	Hypoplastic (inferior portion), occasionally slightly rotated	Normal or slightly enlarged	Normal	Absent	No

Abbreviations: BPC, blake pouch cyst; IVH, isolated vermian hypoplasia; MCM, mega cisterna magna; PFAC, posterior fossa arachnoid cyst.

Rhombencephalosynapsis

Rhombencephalosynapsis is defined by complete or partial absence of the vermis with fusion of the cerebellar hemispheres, dentate nuclei, and cerebellar peduncles.[12] The genetic basis of this malformation is unknown. However, a dorsoventral patterning defect in the rostral midline regions of rhombomere 1 is suspected.[2,3] Affected children present with signs of cerebellar dysfunction, including ataxia, abnormal eye movements, head stereotypies, and delayed motor development. Rhombencephalosynapsis is sporadic, and most of the patients are nonsyndromic. However, it may also occur in the setting of Gomez-Lopez-Hernandez syndrome (parietal alopecia, trigeminal anesthesia, and craniofacial dysmorphic signs) or VACTERL (Vertebral anomalies, Anal atresia, Cardiac defects, Tracheoesophageal fistula and/or Esophageal atresia, Renal anomalies, and Limb defects) association.[1–4,13]

The key neuroimaging findings are as follows (Fig. 4)[12–14]:

- Complete or partial absence of the vermis
- Fusion of the cerebellar hemispheres across the midline with cerebellar folia extending horizontally across the midline
- Fused superior cerebellar peduncles (SCP) and dentate nuclei
- Keyhole-shaped fourth ventricle
- Absence of the vermian primary fissure on midsagittal MR images

Of note, a variable degree of vermian formation and cerebellar hemisphere separation may be present (partial forms).

Supratentorial anomalies include the following[12–14]:

- Midline fusion of the colliculi (mesencephalosynapsis)
- Fused thalami (diencephalosynapsis)
- Hydrocephalus due to aqueductal stenosis/cerebrospinal fluid circulation disorder
- Corpus callosum dysgenesis
- Septum pellucidum agenesis
- Holoprosencephaly (rare)

Cerebellar hypoplasia and dysplasia

A malformed cerebellum may be hypoplastic (reduced cerebellar volume), dysplastic (abnormal cerebellar foliation, fissuration, and white matter architecture), or hypodysplastic (combined hypoplasia and dysplasia).[5] Each part of the cerebellum may be affected, resulting in global or partial cerebellar involvement. The clinical presentation is highly variable and mostly depends on the underlying disease.

On imaging, cerebellar dysplasia is characterized by variable combinations of the following (Fig. 5):

- Abnormal cerebellar foliation/fissuration, including defective, large, or vertical fissures (clefts), abnormal white matter arborization, and blurred gray-white matter interface
- Gray matter heterotopia within the cerebellar white matter
- Cortical thickening, resulting in an irregularly smooth, bumpy cerebellar surface
- Cortical-subcortical cysts usually isointense with cerebrospinal fluid (CSF) in all MR imaging sequences, varying in size, shape, and distribution[15]

Multiple genetic or acquired mechanisms are linked to cerebellar dysplasia, causing disruption of precursor cell division, neuronal migration, cortical layering, and fissure formation. Cerebellar dysplasia is therefore a nonspecific feature associated with several different conditions, such as Poretti-Boltshauser and

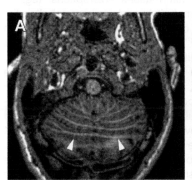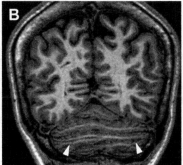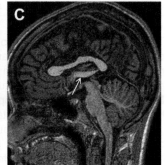

Fig. 4. Rhombencephalosynapsis. (*A*) Axial and (*B*) coronal-reformatted 3-dimensional (3D) T1-weighted MR images demonstrate absence of the vermis and fusion of the cerebellar hemispheres with characteristic uninterrupted horizontal extension of the cerebellar fissures and white matter across the midline (*arrowheads*). (*C*) Sagittal-reformatted 3D T1-weighted MR image reveals lack of definition of the normal vermian lobules resulting in a "cerebellar–not vermian–configuration." Note the low-lying fused fornices (*arrow*).

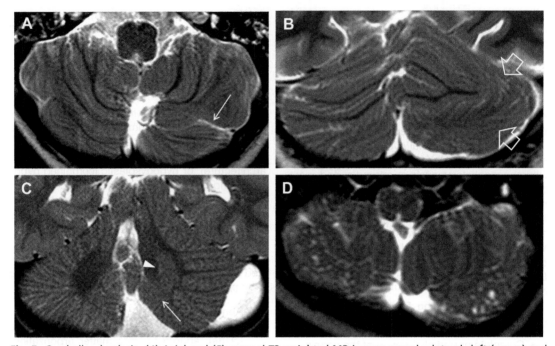

Fig. 5. Cerebellar dysplasia. (*A*) Axial and (*B*) coronal T2-weighted MR images reveal a lateral cleft (*arrow*) and abnormal cerebellar foliation and fissuration with loss of the normal white matter architecture (*open arrows*) in the left cerebellar hemispheres. (*C*) Coronal T2-weighted image reveals blurred gray-white matter interface (*arrow*) with gray matter heterotopia within the cerebellar white matter (*arrowhead*). (*D*) Axial T2-weighted MR image demonstrates bilateral abnormal foliation associated with multiple cortical-subcortical cysts.

Chudley-McCullogh syndromes (**Figs. 6** and **7, Table 3**).[16–20] Additional supratentorial findings are usually helpful to differentiate between the causative diseases (**Fig. 8**). However, in most cases, the exact pathogenesis remains unknown. Of note, unilateral cerebellar hypodysplasia is frequently the result of disruptive events, including prenatal/perinatal cerebellar hemorrhagic or ischemic infarcts, such as in preterm newborns or PHACE syndrome.[21]

Cerebellar and Brainstem Malformations

Pontocerebellar hypoplasia

The term "pontocerebellar hypoplasia" (PCH) is often used in a descriptive manner to refer to a reduction in volume of both cerebellum and pons. However, as conceptualized by Peter Barth, this term has been adopted to indicate a heterogeneous group of prenatal-onset neurodegenerative disorders, mainly but not exclusively affecting the cerebellum and pons.[22] To date, 11 subtypes of PCH with different phenotypes and pathogeneses have been identified (**Table 4**).[22,23] Of note, types 3, 8, and 11 have a nonprogressive course.

Characteristic MR imaging findings are listed as follows (**Fig. 9**):

- Cerebellar hypoplasia with superimposed atrophy
- Absence or significant reduction of the pontine prominence
- Normal or slightly reduced posterior fossa size
- Variable cerebral involvement, including atrophy and delayed myelination

The morphologic pattern of "pontocerebellar hypoplasia" is not specific to PCH: it has been shown in several malformations, disruptions (eg, in extreme prematurity), and neurometabolic diseases (eg, in congenital disorder of glycosylation type 1A).[21–28] In particular, severe cerebellar hypoplasia with pontine hypoplasia is frequently described in patients with mutations in the CASK, RELN, and VLDLR genes.

CASK encodes a multidomain scaffolding protein that regulates expression of genes involved in cortical development, such as RELN.[24] CASK mutations are inherited with an X-linked pattern, occur de novo, and more commonly affect female children, presumably because it is lethal in male children. Affected children present with ataxia, nystagmus, postnatal microcephaly, severe cognitive impairment, seizures, retinopathy, sensorineural hearing loss, and (inconsistently)

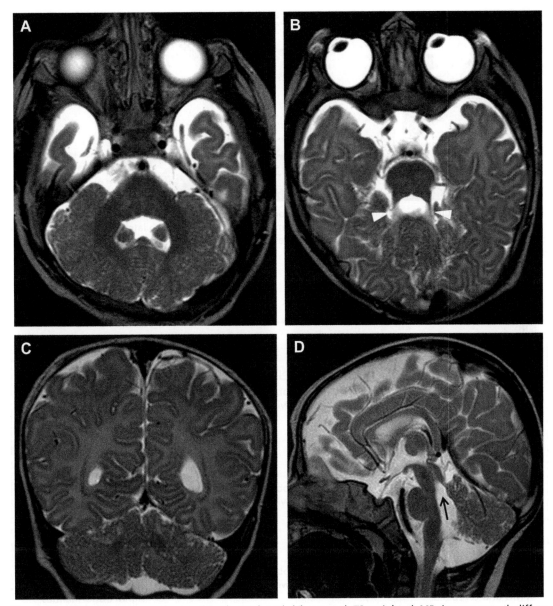

Fig. 6. Poretti-Boltshauser syndrome. (*A*, *B*) Axial and (*C*) coronal T2-weighted MR images reveal diffuse abnormal foliation with multiple cortical-subcortical cysts and thin splayed SCP (molar tooth-like sign, *arrowheads*). (*D*) Midsagittal T2-weighted image shows an enlarged, elongated, and squarelike fourth ventricle (*arrow*). The cerebral cortex is normal.

cataract.[24] The neuroimaging findings include the following (see **Fig. 9**):

- Microcephaly with simplified gyral pattern
- Severe global cerebellar hypoplasia
- Pontine hypoplasia
- Normal-sized corpus callosum[24]

RELN encodes an extracellular matrix–associated glycoprotein (reelin) that is critical for the regulation of neuronal migration during cortical and cerebellar development.[25] Affected children show severe developmental disabilities, microcephaly, seizures, and congenital lymphedema. VLDLR encodes the very-low-density lipoprotein receptor, which acts as a coreceptor for the reelin pathway. VLDLR-associated disorder is characterized by nonprogressive cerebellar ataxia, moderate to profound intellectual disability, dysarthria, strabismus, and seizures.[26] In patients with RELN-related and VLDLR-related disorders, pachygyria

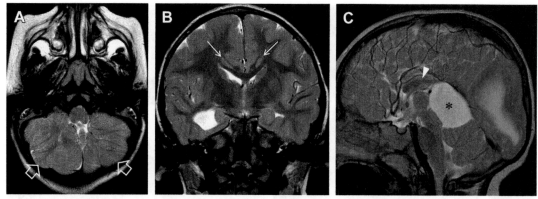

Fig. 7. Chudley-McCullough syndrome. (*A*) Axial, (*B*) coronal, and (*C*) sagittal T2-weighted MR images demonstrate abnormal foliation involving the cerebellar hemispheres (*open arrows*), bilateral cingulate subcortical gray matter heterotopia (*arrows*), partial callosal agenesis (*arrowhead*), and an arachnoid cyst in the quadrigeminal plate cistern (*asterisk*).

Table 3
Clinicoradiological features of genetic cerebellar dysplasias

Disease	Genes	Dysplasia Pattern	Associated Features
Alpha dystroglycanopathies	>15 genes	Global cerebellar dysplasia with multiple cysts	CMD, increased CK level, cobblestone malformation, supratentorial WM signal abnormalities, brainstem kinking, eye involvement
LAMB1-related cobblestone malformation	LAMB1	Global cerebellar dysplasia with multiple cysts	Variable muscular or ocular abnormalities, cobblestone malformation, supratentorial WM signal abnormalities
GPR56-related and COL3A1-related PMG and cerebellar dysplasia	GPR56, COL3A1	Global cerebellar dysplasia with multiple cysts	Bifrontal PMG, supratentorial WM signal abnormalities
Poretti-Boltshauser syndrome	LAMA1	Global cerebellar dysplasia with multiple cysts	Myopia, retinal abnormality
Chudley-McCullough syndrome	GPSM2	Abnormal foliation/ fissuration inferior hemispheres	Hearing loss, frontal and cingulate PMG/ heterotopia, partial callosal agenesis
Tubulinopathies	TUBA1A, TUBA8, TUBB2A, TUBB2B, TUBB3, TUBB5, TUBG1	Diagonal folia across vermis	Dysmorphic basal ganglia, cortical malformations, callosal dysgenesis, asymmetric brainstem
Joubert Syndrome (Ciliopathy)	>30 genes	Dysplastic superior and hypoplastic inferior vermis and hemispheres	Molar tooth sign, variably associated supratentorial malformations

Abbreviations: CK, creatine kinase; CMD, congenital muscular dystrophy; WM, white matter.

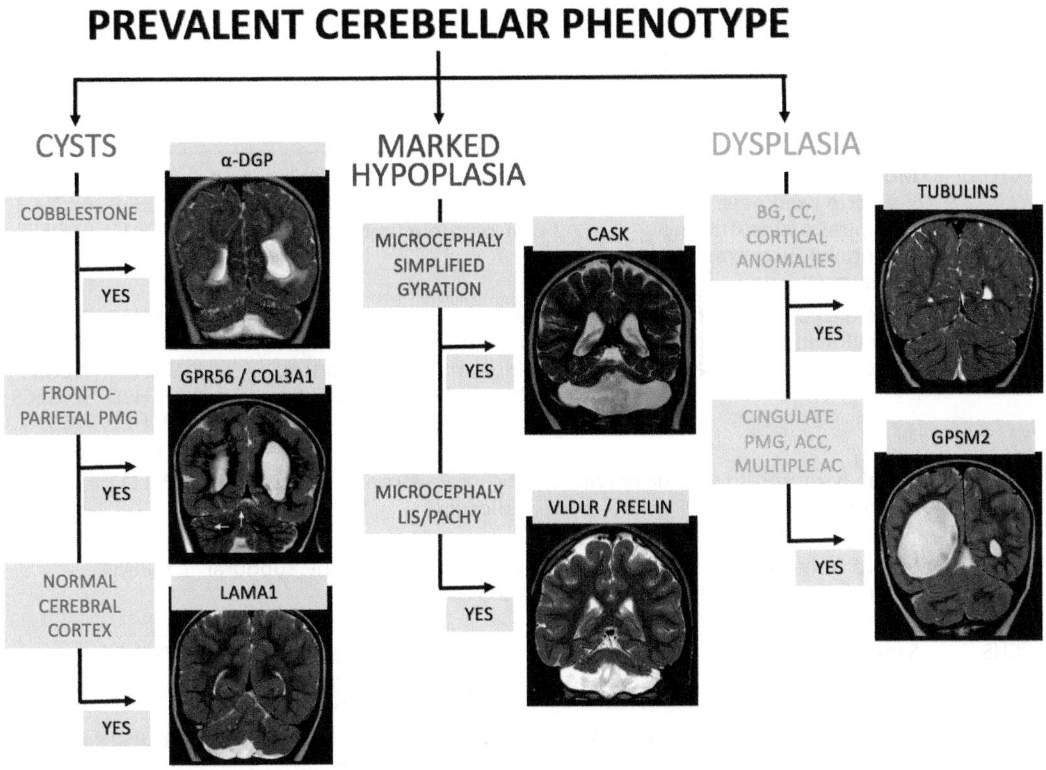

PREVALENT CEREBELLAR PHENOTYPE

Fig. 8. Graphic flowchart for reviewing MR imaging scans displaying sigs of cerebellar dysplasia. AC, arachnoid cyst; ACC, agenesis of the corpus callosum; BG, basal ganglia; CC, corpus callosum; CASK, calcium/calmodulin-dependent serine protein kinase gene; COL3A1, collagen, type III, alpha-1 gene; GPR56, G protein-coupled receptor 56 gene; GPSM2, G Protein Signaling Modulator 2 gene; LAMA1, Laminin Subunit Alpha 1 gene; VLDLR, Very Low Density Lipoprotein Receptor gene; α-DGP, alpha-dystroglycanopathies.

(more severe in patients with RELN mutations) and extreme cerebellar hypoplasia with absent cerebellar folia and preferential vermian involvement (especially in VLDLR mutations) are characteristic neuroimaging features (see **Fig. 9**).[5,26]

Finally, PCH is found in congenital muscular dystrophies, resulting from mutations in genes responsible for the O-glycosylation and rarely N-glycosylation of alpha-dystroglycans.[27] Recessive mutations in these genes cause overlapping phenotypes characterized by muscular (weakness, hypotonia, and increased creatine kinase values), cerebral (intellectual disability, seizures, and tetraspasticity), and ocular (microphthalmia, optic nerve hypoplasia, chorioretinal coloboma, cataract, glaucoma, or high myopia) involvement. Based on the severity of the findings, different phenotypes have been described (in order of increasing severity): Fukuyama congenital muscular dystrophy, muscle-eye-brain disease, and Walker-Warburg syndrome.[27]

Infratentorial neuroimaging findings include the following (**Fig. 10**):

- Pontocerebellar hypoplasia
- Cerebellar dysplasia with subcortical cysts

- Dysplastic tectum
- Ventral pontine cleft
- Brainstem kinking

Supratentorial findings comprise the following:

- Mild ventriculomegaly to severe hydrocephalus
- White matter abnormalities/hypomyelination
- Cobblestone cortex[27]

Tubulinopathies

Tubulinopathies are a group of brain malformations caused by mutations of α- and β-tubulin genes (see **Table 3**).[20,28,29] Most of these mutations are de novo without risk of recurrence. Children present with variable degrees of intellectual disability, tetraspastic cerebral palsy, postnatal microcephaly, and early-onset therapy-resistant seizures. Dysmorphic features are rare, and other organs are not affected.

The spectrum of posterior fossa abnormalities includes the following (**Fig. 11**)[20,28,29]:

- Different degrees of PCH
- Cerebellar dysplasia with typical diagonal hemispheric cleft involving the superior vermis

Table 4
Pontocerebellar hypoplasia subtypes

Subtype	Clinical Features	Neuroimaging Features Associated with PCH	Subcategory and Gene
PCH1	Motor neuron degeneration, muscle weakness, hypotonia, respiratory insufficiency, congenital contractures, early death	Variable pontine involvement, CC hypoplasia, cortical atrophy, incomplete myelination	PCH1A: VRK1 PCH1B: EXOSC3 PCH1C: EXOSC8 PCH1D: SLC25A46
PCH2	Generalized clonus, impaired swallowing, dystonia, chorea, progressive microcephaly	Involvement hemispheres >> vermis (dragonfly appearance), hemispheric cavitations, cerebral atrophy	PCH2A: TSEN54 PCH2B: TSEN2 PCH2C: TSEN34 PCH2D: SEPSECS PCH2E: VPS53 PCH2F: TSEN15
PCH3	Facial dysmorphisms, optic nerve atrophy, progressive microcephaly	Optic nerve atrophy, thin corpus callosum	PCLO
PCH4	Severe form of PCH2 with congenital contractures, microcephaly, polyhydramnios	Severe cerebral atrophy, subdural fluid collections	TSEN54
PCH5	Same as PCH4	Severe cerebral atrophy, subdural fluid collections, involvement vermis >> hemispheres	TSEN54
PCH6	Hypotonia, seizures, elevated CSF lactate	Rapidly progressive supratentorial and infratentorial atrophy	RARS2
PCH7	Disorder of sexual development	Severe WM reduction, enlarged ventricles	TOE1
PCH8	Abnormal muscle tone, dystonia, ataxia, no/little progression	Proportionate involvement of vermis and hemispheres, nonprogressive course	CHMP1A
PCH9	Abnormal muscle tone, impaired swallowing, progressive microcephaly	Callosal dysgenesis, "figure-of-8" midbrain appearance, small hyperintense basal ganglia, and hypointense thalami	AMPD2
PCH10	Abnormal muscle tone, seizures, motor neuron degeneration, microcephaly	Mild cerebellar hypoplasia/atrophy, thin corpus callosum, myelination delay	CLP1
PCH11	severe neurodevelopmental delay, microcephaly, hypotonia	Nonprogressive PCH, callosal hypoplasia	TBC1D23

- Asymmetric midbrain and pons with clefts
- Asymmetric cerebral peduncles

Characteristic supratentorial findings are as follows[20,28,29]:

- Cortical malformations (lissencephaly, polymicrogyria, and dysgyria)
- Dysmorphic basal ganglia due to internal capsule anomalies
- Dysmorphic ventriculomegaly
- Agenesis/dysgenesis of the corpus callosum and anterior commissure

DTI and FT studies may reveal axonal pathfinding anomalies, including anterior commissure absence, abnormal callosal connectivity, reduced transverse pontine fibers with slanting course, and small asymmetric corticospinal tracts.[20,28,29]

Joubert syndrome

Joubert syndrome refers to a group of rare conditions, also called ciliopathies, that stem from defects in a cellular organelle, the primary nonmotile cilium. Primary cilia play a key role in the development and functioning of various cells, including

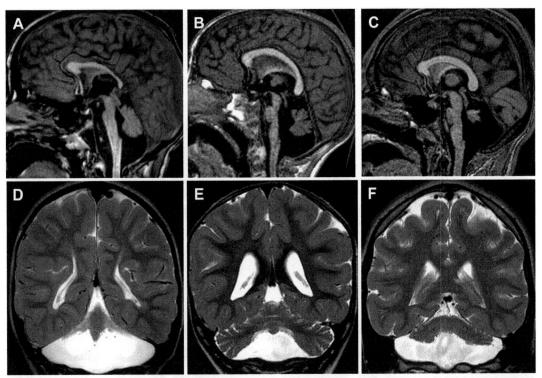

Fig. 9. PCHs. PCH 2: (*A*) midsagittal T1-weighted and (*D*) coronal T2-weighted MR images reveal marked hypoplasia of the pons and cerebellum with more severe involvement of the cerebellar hemispheres relative to the vermis ("dragonfly" appearance). Callosal hypoplasia is also noted. CASK-related PCH: (*B*) midsagittal T1-weighted and (*E*) coronal T2-weighted MR images demonstrate hypoplasia of the pons and cerebellum with proportionate involvement of the cerebellar hemispheres relative to the vermis. The signal intensity of the cerebellar hemispheres is normal (in contrast with PCH 2). Microcephaly with simplified gyral pattern is also noted. VLDLR-related PCH: (*C*) midsagittal T1-weighted and (*F*) coronal T2-weighted MR images show hypoplasia of the pons and cerebellum with typical absence of cerebellar foliation and preferential vermian involvement. Note the associated lissencephaly.

retinal photoreceptors, epithelial cells lining the renal tubules, bile ducts, and neurons.[30,31] In the CNS, they are implicated in neuronal cell proliferation and axonal migration in the cerebellum and brainstem. Ciliopathies are characterized by an extreme genetic heterogeneity, with more than 30 genes identified so far. Mutations in all these genes but OFD1 are autosomal recessively inherited, resulting in a recurrence risk of 25%.[30,31] Affected patients typically present with ocular (colobomas, retinal dystrophy), hepatic (congenital hepatic fibrosis), skeletal (different forms of polydactyly), and renal (nephronophthisis) abnormalities. Common neurologic symptoms include hypotonia, breathing abnormalities, variable intellectual disability, ataxia, and ocular motor apraxia.[30] The "molar tooth sign" observed on axial neuroimaging is required for the diagnosis and is defined by elongated, thickened, and horizontally orientated SCP, a deep interpeduncular fossa, and vermian hypoplasia (Fig. 12).[30–32] Of

note, the degree of vermian hypoplasia, shape of the "molar tooth," size of the posterior fossa, and degree of cerebellar hypodysplasia are variable. Brainstem abnormalities are present in about 30% of cases, including a dysmorphic tectum and midbrain, thickened and elongated midbrain, and small pons.[32] Supratentorial anomalies are detected in about 30% of cases:

- Callosal dysgenesis
- Encephaloceles
- Hypothalamic hamartomas (in oral facial digital syndrome type VI)
- Cortical malformations
- Ventriculomegaly

Differences in neuroimaging findings can be present within siblings representing an intrafamilial heterogeneity.[32] Except for oral facial digital syndrome type VI, no neuroimaging-genotype correlations are known. DTI reveals underlying defects of axonal guidance, including lack of

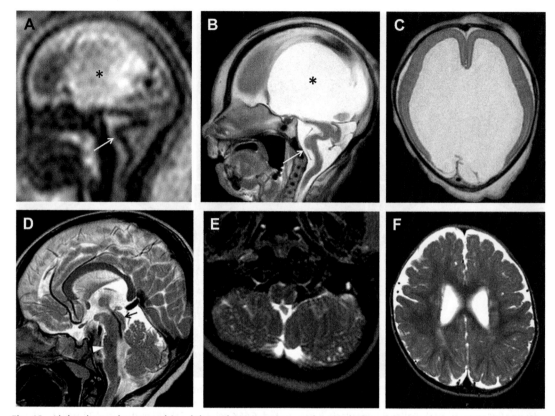

Fig. 10. Alpha-dystroglycanopathies. (*A*) Fetal MR imaging, midsagittal T2-weighted image, and (*B, C*) matching postmortem midsagittal and axial T2-weighted MR images, performed in a fetus with Walker-Warburg syndrome (21 gestational weeks), demonstrate severe supratentorial hydrocephalus (*asterisks*) with marked kinking of the brainstem (*arrows*). (*D*) Sagittal and (*E*) axial T2-weighted MR images in a child with muscle-eye-brain disease show a dysplastic midbrain and tectum (*arrow*), a thinned pons (*arrowhead*), multiple bilateral subcortical cysts in the cerebellar hemispheres, mild ventriculomegaly, multifocal white matter changes, and cobblestone malformation (*F*).

SCP decussation,[6] abnormal corticospinal tracts course (decaying molar tooth),[33] and ectopic transverse white matter tracts in the ventral midbrain (anterior mesencephalic cap dysplasia).[34]

Predominant Brainstem Malformations

Pontine tegmental cap dysplasia
Pontine tegmental cap dysplasia is a rare sporadic brainstem malformation with unknown genotype and no familial recurrence.[35] Clinically, it is characterized by cranial nerve deficits (including hearing loss, facial paralysis, trigeminal anesthesia, and dysphagia), cognitive disability, and ataxia. The degree of brainstem dysplasia grossly correlates with the developmental disability. Vertebral segmentation anomalies, rib malformations, and congenital heart defects have also been observed.

Neuroimaging findings include the following[7,35,36] (**Fig. 13**):

- Ventral pons flattening
- A vaulted pontine tegmentum (the cap)
- Small asymmetric middle cerebellar peduncles
- Inferior cerebellar peduncles agenesis
- Vermian hypoplasia
- Molar toothlike aspect of the ponto-mesencephalic junction
- Absent inferior olivary prominence
- Duplicated internal auditory canals
- Hypoplastic cranial nerves

DTI shows absence of the transverse pontine fibers and SCP decussation, and presence of a transverse axonal band at the level of the "cap" along the dorsal pons.[4,7]

Horizontal gaze palsy with progressive scoliosis
Horizontal gaze palsy with progressive scoliosis is a rare autosomal recessive disorder caused by

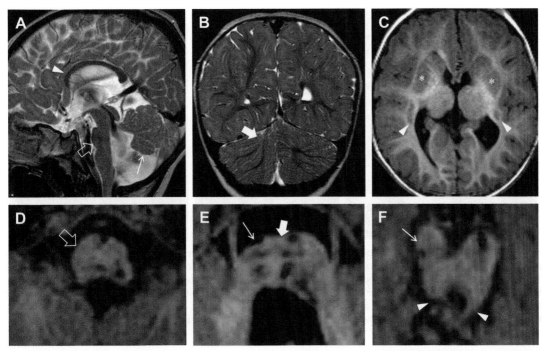

Fig. 11. Tubulinopathy. (A) Sagittal and (B) coronal T2-weighted MR images reveal callosal hypo-dysgenesis (*arrowhead*), pontine hypoplasia (*open arrow*), a smaller and slightly upward rotated vermis (*arrow*), and right unilateral cerebellar dysplasia with oblique folia (*thick arrow*). (C) Axial 3D T1-weighted MR image demonstrates dysmorphic basal ganglia (*asterisks*), diffuse dysgyria, and subcortical gray matter heterotopias (*arrowheads*). (D–F) Axial color-coded FA maps overlaid to axial 3D T1-weighted images, magnified views, show enlargement of the right portion of medulla (*open arrow*), pontine, and midbrain asymmetry with smaller right corticospinal tract (*arrows*), reduced anterior transverse pontine fibers (*thick arrow*), and dysmorphic SCP (*arrowheads*).

mutations in ROBO3, encoding a receptor required for axonal guidance.[37–39] Affected children have congenital absence of horizontal eye movements, preservation of vertical gaze and convergence, and progressive scoliosis. Neurocognitive functions are typically preserved.[37–39]

Neuroimaging findings include the following (Fig. 14):

- A butterfly-shaped medulla, due to the missing prominence of the gracile and cuneate nuclei

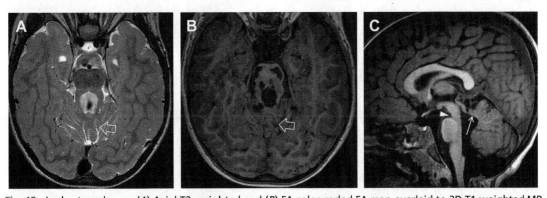

Fig. 12. Joubert syndrome. (A) Axial T2-weighted and (B) FA color-coded FA map overlaid to 3D T1-weighted MR images show the molar tooth sign characterized by elongated, thickened, and horizontally oriented SCP and a deep interpeduncular fossa. (C) Sagittal T1-weighted MR image reveals hypoplasia and dysplasia of the vermis (*open arrow*), enlargement of the fourth ventricle with upward and posterior displacement of the fastigium (*arrow*), and a narrow pontomesencephalic isthmus (*arrowhead*).

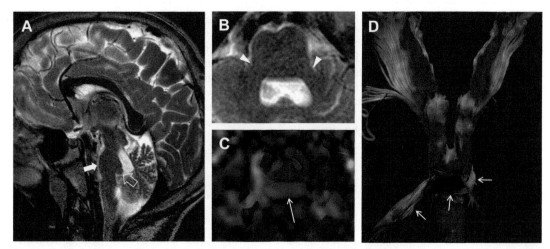

Fig. 13. Pontine tegmental cap dysplasia. (*A*) Midsagittal T2-weighted image demonstrates a flattened ventral pons (*arrow*), a cap covering the dorsal pons and protruding into the fourth ventricle (*open arrow*). (*B*) Axial T2-weighted and (*C*) and FA color-coded FA map overlaid to 3D T1-weighted MR images show bilateral hypoplastic MCP (*arrowheads*), absence of the normal pontocerebellar transverse fibers, and an aberrant dorsal transverse axonal band at the level of the cap along the dorsal pons (*arrow*). (*D*) FT reconstruction, posterior view, reveals the misoriented fibers connecting the basal pons to the cerebellar hemisphere through the MCP (*arrows*).

- Pontine hypoplasia with dorsal midline cleft
- Absence of the facial colliculi bulging contour
- Prominence of inferior olivary nuclei

DTI typically shows absence of the decussation of corticospinal tracts, pontine sensory tracts, and SCP.[5,39]

Diencephalic-mesencephalic junction dysplasia
Diencephalic-mesencephalic junction dysplasia is characterized by dorsoventral enlargement and abnormal butterfly-like contour of the midbrain on axial sections.[40] Clinical features include cognitive impairment, axial hypotonia, spastic tetraparesis, and seizures. Recently, mutations in the protocadherin-12 gene, encoding a cell surface protein promoting cell adhesion and neurite outgrowth, have been identified in some of these patients.[41] Additional features include ventriculomegaly, PCH, calcifications, and abnormalities of the corticospinal tracts, commissures, basal ganglia, and olfactory bulbs.[42,43] Recently, the

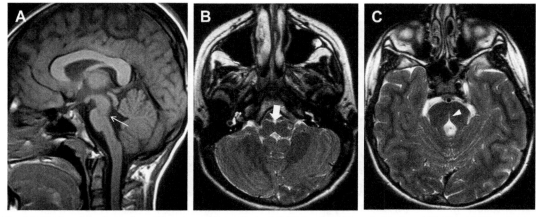

Fig. 14. Horizontal gaze palsy with progressive scoliosis. (*A*) Midsagittal T1-weighted and (*B, C*) axial T2-weighted MR images show depression of the floor of the fourth ventricle (*arrow*), a butterfly medulla with more prominent inferior olivary nuclei compared with the pyramids (*thick arrow*), and a deep dorsal midline pontine cleft (*arrowhead*).

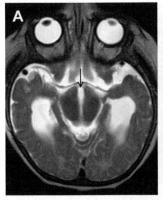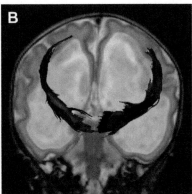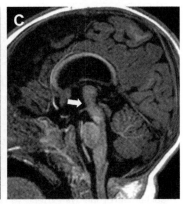

Fig. 15. Diencephalic-mesencephalic junction dysplasia (DMJD). (A) Axial T2-weighted MR image of a child with type A DMJD shows fusion of the hypothalamus and midbrain, enlargement of the dorsoventral axis of the midbrain, and ventral midbrain cleft (arrow) resulting in a butterfly-like appearance. (B) FT superimposed to a coronal T2-weighted MR image reveals abrupt interruption of the corticospinal tracts at the level of the midbrain in another patient with type A DMJD. (C) Sagittal 3D T1-weighted MR image demonstrates fusion of the midbrain with the interthalamic mass (arrow) in a patient with type B DMJD.

spectrum of diencephalic-mesencephalic junction anomalies has expanded, including the following (Fig. 15):

- Type A forms with complete hypothalamic-mesencephalic fusion leading to dorsoventral enlargement and abnormal contour of the midbrain on axial planes, variably associated with a ventral cleft or linear T2-hyperintensities.
- Type B forms are characterized by incomplete cleavage between the thalami and the mesencephalon on the sagittal plane, variably associated with brainstem and/or vermian hypoplasia.

DTI shows an abrupt arrest of corticospinal tracts at the level of the diencephalon, suggesting disturbed axonal path-finding.[40,42]

SUMMARY

Posterior fossa malformations represent a wide variety of disorders that may involve different parts of the pons and cerebellum. Neuroimaging plays a key role in the diagnosis of these conditions with well-defined neuroimaging-based diagnostic criteria. Accurate classification of cerebellar and brainstem malformations is important for therapy, prognosis, and genetic counseling. In addition, advanced neuroimaging, including DTI and FT, may provide important information about the pathogenesis, serving as a biomarker for cognitive outcome in selected cerebellar and brainstem malformations.

ACKNOWLEDGMENTS

This work was supported by funds from Current Research for the 2018-2020 triennium – Research Line 5 on Muscular and Neurological Disorders – Ministry of Health—Italy.

REFERENCES

1. Barkovich AJ, Millen KJ, Dobyns WB. A developmental and genetic classification for midbrain-hindbrain malformations. Brain 2009; 132(Pt 12):3199–230.
2. Doherty D, Millen KJ, Barkovich AJ. Midbrain and hindbrain malformations: advances in clinical diagnosis, imaging, and genetics. Lancet Neurol 2013; 12(4):381–93.
3. Poretti A, Boltshauser E, Huisman TA. Cerebellar and brainstem malformations. Neuroimaging Clin N Am 2016;26(3):341–57.
4. Jissendi-Tchofo P, Severino M, Nguema-Edzang B, et al. Update on neuroimaging phenotypes of mid-hindbrain malformations. Neuroradiology 2015; 57(2):113–38.
5. Poretti A, Meoded A, Rossi A, et al. Diffusion tensor imaging and fiber tractography in brain malformations. Pediatr Radiol 2013;43(1):28–54.
6. Poretti A, Boltshauser E, Loenneker T, et al. Diffusion tensor imaging in Joubert syndrome. AJNR Am J Neuroradiol 2007;28(10):1929–33.
7. Jissendi-Tchofo P, Doherty D, McGillivray G, et al. Pontine tegmental cap dysplasia: MR imaging and diffusion tensor imaging features of impaired axonal navigation. AJNR Am J Neuroradiol 2009;30(1):113–9.
8. Garel C. Posterior fossa malformations: main features and limits in prenatal diagnosis. Pediatr Radiol 2010;40(6):1038–45.
9. Aldinger KA, Lehmann OJ, Hudgins L, et al. FOXC1 is required for normal cerebellar development and is a

major contributor to chromosome 6p25.3 Dandy-Walker malformation. Nat Genet 2009;41(9):1037–42.

10. Alexiou GA, Sfakianos G, Prodromou N. Dandy-Walker malformation: analysis of 19 cases. J Child Neurol 2010;25(2):188–91.

11. Correa GG, Amaral LF, Vedolin LM. Neuroimaging of Dandy-Walker malformation: new concepts. Top Magn Reson Imaging 2011;22(6):303–12.

12. Ishak GE, Dempsey JC, Shaw DW, et al. Rhomben-cephalosynapsis: a hindbrain malformation associated with incomplete separation of midbrain and forebrain, hydrocephalus and a broad spectrum of severity. Brain 2012;135(Pt 5):1370–86.

13. Sukhudyan B, Jaladyan V, Melikyan G, et al. Gomez-Lopez-Hernandez syndrome: reappraisal of the diagnostic criteria. Eur J Pediatr 2010;169(12):1523–8.

14. Whitehead MT, Choudhri AF, Grimm J, et al. Rhom-bencephalosynapsis as a cause of aqueductal stenosis: an under-recognized association in hydrocephalic children. Pediatr Radiol 2014;44(7):849–56.

15. Boltshauser E, Scheer I, Huisman TA, et al. Cerebellar cysts in children: a pattern recognition approach. Cerebellum 2015;14(3):308–16.

16. Doherty D, Chudley AE, Coghlan G, et al. GPSM2 mutations cause the brain malformations and hearing loss in Chudley-McCullough syndrome. Am J Hum Genet 2012;90(6):1088–93.

17. Bahi-Buisson N, Poirier K, Boddaert N, et al. GPR56-related bilateral frontoparietal polymicrogyria: further evidence for an overlap with the cobblestone complex. Brain 2010;133(11):3194–209.

18. Vandervore L, Stouffs K, Tanyalçin I, et al. Bi-allelic variants in COL3A1 encoding the ligand to GPR56 are associated with cobblestone-like cortical malformation, white matter changes and cerebellar cysts. J Med Genet 2017;54(6):432–40.

19. Micalizzi A, Poretti A, Romani M, et al. Clinical, neuroradiological and molecular characterization of cerebellar dysplasia with cysts (Poretti-Boltshauser syndrome). Eur J Hum Genet 2016;24(9):1262–7.

20. Romaniello R, Arrigoni F, Panzeri E, et al. Tubulin-related cerebellar dysplasia: definition of a distinct pattern of cerebellar malformation. Eur Radiol 2017;27(12):5080–92.

21. Poretti A, Boltshauser E, Huisman TA. Prenatal cerebellar disruptions: neuroimaging spectrum of findings in correlation with likely mechanisms and etiologies of injury. Neuroimaging Clin N Am 2016;26(3):359–72.

22. van Dijk T, Baas F, Barth PG, et al. What's new in pontocerebellar hypoplasia? An update on genes and subtypes. Orphanet J Rare Dis 2018;13(1):92.

23. Accogli A, Iacomino M, Pinto F, et al. Novel AMPD2 mutation in pontocerebellar hypoplasia, dysmorphisms, and teeth abnormalities. Neurol Genet 2017;3(5):e179.

24. Burglen L, Chantot-Bastaraud S, Garel C, et al. Spectrum of pontocerebellar hypoplasia in 13 girls and boys with CASK mutations: confirmation of a recognizable phenotype and first description of a male mosaic patient. Orphanet J Rare Dis 2012;7:18.

25. Hong SE, Shugart YY, Huang DT, et al. Autosomal recessive lissencephaly with cerebellar hypoplasia is associated with human RELN mutations. Nat Genet 2000;26(1):93–6.

26. Valence S, Garel C, Barth M, et al. RELN and VLDLR mutations underlie two distinguishable clinico-radiological phenotypes. Clin Genet 2016;90(6):545–9.

27. Clement E, Mercuri E, Godfrey C, et al. Brain involvement in muscular dystrophies with defective dystroglycan glycosylation. Ann Neurol 2008;64(5):573–82.

28. Romaniello R, Arrigoni F, Cavallini A, et al. Brain malformations and mutations in alpha- and beta-tubulin genes: a review of the literature and description of two new cases. Dev Med Child Neurol 2014;56(4):354–60.

29. Arrigoni F, Romaniello R, Peruzzo D, et al. The spectrum of brainstem malformations associated to mutations of the tubulin genes family: MRI and DTI analysis. Eur Radiol 2019;29(2):770–82.

30. Romani M, Micalizzi A, Valente EM. Joubert syndrome: congenital cerebellar ataxia with the molar tooth. Lancet Neurol 2013;12(9):894–905.

31. Hildebrandt F, Benzing T, Katsanis N. Ciliopathies. N Engl J Med 2011;364(16):1533–43.

32. Poretti A, Snow J, Summers AC, et al. Joubert syndrome: neuroimaging findings in 110 patients in correlation with cognitive function and genetic cause. J Med Genet 2017;54(8):521–9.

33. Alves CAPF, Ferraciolli S, Matsui C, et al. Decaying molar tooth sign in Joubert syndrome and related disorders is correlated to a displacement of the corticospinal tract. Neuroradiology 2017;59(12):1189–91.

34. Arrigoni F, Romaniello R, Peruzzo D, et al. Anterior mesencephalic cap dysplasia: novel brain stem malformative features associated with Joubert syndrome. AJNR Am J Neuroradiol 2017;38(12):2385–90.

35. Barth PG, Majoie CB, Caan MW, et al. Pontine tegmental cap dysplasia: a novel brain malformation with a defect in axonal guidance. Brain 2007;130(Pt 9):2258–66.

36. Desai NK, Young L, Miranda MA, et al. Pontine tegmental cap dysplasia: the neurotologic perspective. Otolaryngol Head Neck Surg 2011;145(6):992–8.

37. Bosley TM, Salih MA, Jen JC, et al. Neurologic features of horizontal gaze palsy and progressive scoliosis with mutations in ROBO3. Neurology 2005; 64(7):1196–203.

38. Rossi A, Catala M, Biancheri R, et al. MR imaging of brain-stem hypoplasia in horizontal gaze palsy with progressive scoliosis. AJNR Am J Neuroradiol 2004;25(6):1046–8.

39. Haller S, Wetzel SG, Lutschg J. Functional MRI, DTI and neurophysiology in horizontal gaze palsy with progressive scoliosis. Neuroradiology 2008;50(5): 453–9.

40. Zaki MS, Saleem SN, Dobyns WB, et al. Diencephalic-mesencephalic junction dysplasia: a novel recessive brain malformation. Brain 2012;135(Pt 8): 2416–27.

41. Guemez-Gamboa A, Çağlayan AO, Stanley V, et al. Loss of protocadherin-12 leads to diencephalic-mesencephalic junction dysplasia syndrome. Ann Neurol 2018;84(5):638–47.

42. Severino M, Tortora D, Pistorio A, et al. Expanding the spectrum of congenital anomalies of the diencephalic-mesencephalic junction. Neuroradiology 2016;58(1):33–44.

43. Severino M, Righini A, Tortora D, et al. MR imaging diagnosis of diencephalic-mesencephalic junction dysplasia in fetuses with developmental ventriculomegaly. AJNR Am J Neuroradiol 2017;38(8):1643–6.

The Distal Spine
Normal Embryogenesis and Derangements Leading to Malformation

Thomas P. Naidich, MD[a,*], Javin Schefflein, MD[a], Mario A. Cedillo, MD[a],
Jacob P. Deutsch, MD[a], Shashidhara Murthy, MD[a], Mary Fowkes, MD, PhD[b]

KEYWORDS

- Spinal column • Spinal cord • Spinal embryogenesis • Spinal malformations • Axis extension
- Somitogenesis • Junctional neurulation

KEY POINTS

- Concentration gradients of signaling molecules may induce, reinforce or repress secondary programs that lead to differing cell and tissue fates, immediately or after long delay.
- The four paralogous Hox gene clusters determine segment identity through temporal and spatial colinearity, posterior induction, and posterior prevalence.
- The stem cell population maintained in the tailbud provides the "raw material" for axis elongation and formation of the caudal body, spinal column and cord.
- The spinal cord is formed by 3 mechanisms: primary neurulation anteriorly, secondary neurulation posteriorly and junctional neurulation in the middle.
- Delta-Notch-synchronized gene oscillations interact with gradients of FGF, RA and Wnt to induce Tbx6, Mesp2 and Ripply1/2 patterning of somite number and position.

INTRODUCTION

The spine and spinal cord are composed of multiple segments initiated by different embryologic mechanisms and advanced under different systems of control. In humans, the upper central nervous system is formed by primary neurulation, the lower by secondary neurulation, and the intervening segment by junctional neurulation. This article focuses on the distal spine and spinal cord to address their embryogenesis and the molecular derangements that lead to some distal spinal malformations.

GLOSSARY OF TERMS

Table 1 summarizes many of the key terms used in this article.

MECHANISMS UNDERLYING EMBRYOGENESIS
Signals and Signaling Gradients

Much of the signaling that governs embryogenesis depends on the establishment of concentration gradients of molecular signals in which different ranges of signal concentration induce, reinforce, or repress secondary programs that lead, in turn, to different cell and tissue fates. These signaling gradients arise at different sites during different phases of embryogenesis. The signals may be encoded very early in embryogenesis and then remain latent within precursor cells for long periods until they become activated in progeny at later stages of development. The same signal system may be reused to achieve a different goal at a later period of development. The molecular signals

Disclosure: The authors have no conflicts of interest concerning the information within or the publication of this article.
[a] Department of Radiology, Icahn School of Medicine at Mt. Sinai, One Gustave Levy Place, New York, NY 10029, USA; [b] Department of Pathology, Icahn School of Medicine at Mt. Sinai, One Gustave Levy Place, New York, NY 10029, USA
* Corresponding author.
E-mail address: thomas.naidich@mountsinai.org

Table 1
Glossary of terms needed to review the mechanisms of embryogenesis of the spine

Term	Definition, Description, Action
β-Catenin	A dual-function protein encoded by the gene *CTNNB1* and involved in cell-cell adhesion and gene transcription. It is an intracellular transducer in the Wnt signaling pathway and forms part of the cadherin protein complex
bHLH	Basic helix-loop-helix, a superfamily known as DNA-binding transcription factors appearing as homodimers
BMPs	Bone morphogenetic proteins, multifunctional growth factors that belong to the TGFβ superfamily. BMPs function in a wide variety of signaling programs. Smad1, Smad5, and Smad8 are the molecules immediately downstream of BMP receptors and play a central role in BMP signal transduction
Brachyury	The gene *brachyury* (short tail) elaborates an embryonic nuclear transcription factor with a conserved role in defining the midline and the anteroposterior axis of the embryo. Previously designated T or Bra, it is now redesignated TBXT
Canonical Wnt/β-catenin signaling	A highly complex signaling cascade in which members of the Wnt family of secreted glycolipoproteins interact with cell surface receptor Frizzled and a coreceptor to stabilize the cytoplasmic protein β-catenin. Increasing levels of β-catenin within the cytoplasm allow it to enter the nucleus, where it acts to derepress Wnt target genes. β-catenin is also a subunit in the cadherin protein complex
Cdx1, Cdx2, Cdx4	Caudal-like homeobox genes that activate Hox genes by chromatin rearrangement. Cdx2 also regulates cyp26a1 to influence RA signal gradients
cyp26a1	Cytochrome p450 26a1 enzyme. This enzyme degrades RA to reduce its concentration and establish a gradient of decreasing RA concentration
Dact1	Disheveled binding antagonist of β-catenin 1
Delta-Notch	A system of cell-cell signaling that enables a dominant cell that carries the Delta ligand to inhibit/regulate the actions of adjacent receiving cells via Notch receptors. Many embryologic systems use Delta-Notch signaling for diverse ends.
Delta/DLL3	Deltalike 3
DSL	*Delta/Serrate/lag-2* family: cell surface molecules that bind to Notch receptors on adjoining cells
Dusp4, Dusp6	Dual-specificity phosphatases 4 and 6 inactivate target kinases by dephosphorylating them at 2 sites
EMT	Epithelial-to-mesenchymal transition; see MET
EphA, EphB	Two different families of membrane-bound protein receptors classified as EphAs or EphBs based on their binding affinity for either the ephrin-A or ephrin-B ligands
Ephrins	Membrane-bound proteins that may serve as ligands for the EphA, EphB, FGF receptors or serve as receptors for other ephrins
ERKs	A family of extracellular signal-regulated kinases
FGF/FGFR	Fibroblast growth factor/fibroblast growth factor receptor. FGFs are a family of polypeptide growth factors that serve as morphogens by acting through 4 FGF receptors Targets of FGF8 include SPRY2, Dusp6, WNT3A and its targets AXIN2, MESGN1, EPHA4, RALDH2, and Paraxis (TCF15)
Foxc1, foxc2	Forkhead box C1 (and C2) genes, involved in the segmentation of paraxial mesoderm and formation of somites. Their expression is graded from low levels caudally to high levels cephalically. Embryos homozygously mutant for both Fox proteins fail to form the uppermost somites: 1–8
Hairy 1, Hairy2	Cyclic (oscillating) genes that establish the segmentation clock. In diverse phyla, similar genes are designated Hairy1 and Hairy2 (in chick), hairy and enhancer of split 1 (Hes1) and Hes7 (in mouse), and Hairy and enhancer of spilt-related 1 (Her1) and Her7 in zebrafish

(*continued on next page*)

Table 1
(continued)

Term	Definition, Description, Action
HER	HES-related transcription factors (see HES)
HES	Members of the *hairy* and *enhancer of split* (*HES*)/*HES-related* (*HER*) genes that are core components of the segmentation (somitogenesis) clock and function mainly as Notch effectors
HDAC1	Histone deacetylase 1
HOX	Homeobox, a DNA sequence of about 180 base pairs found within morphogenic genes that help pattern anatomy. These genes encode homeodomain protein products that serve as transcription factors to help regulate anatomy
HoxD13	The most 5′ gene in the HoxD cluster, associated with termination of axis elongation
LFNG	Lunatic fringe. A somitic clock gene in the chicken and mouse. The fringe family of genes encodes glycosyltransferase enzymes that can modify sugar residues on Notch receptors to alter their binding preferences
Mesp2	Mesoderm posterior 2, a member of the MESP family of transcription factors. They are considered master regulators of the segmentation program that forms the future segment boundaries
MET	Mesenchymal-to-epithelial transition; see EMT
Msgn1	Mesogenin 1. Msgn1 is a *Wnt*-regulated bHLH transcription factor that acts downstream of Wnt3a signaling and upstream or parallel with Tbx6 to promote the maturation of progenitors into mesoderm, rather than neural tissue
mRNA	Messenger RNA
NCAM	Neural cell adhesion molecule
NEUROG3	In humans the NEUROG3 gene encodes Neurogenin-3 protein
Nkx1.2	In humans, a gene on chromosome10q26.13 that encodes a DNA-binding homeobox protein that functions in cell specification, especially in the CNS
Nkx-2.2	In humans, a homeobox protein encoded by NKX2-2 on chromosome 20, likely a nuclear transcription factor. In the developing spinal cord, Nkx-2.2 regulates IRX3, continuing the differentiation of ventral horn neurons
Notch	Part of the Delta-Notch cell-cell signaling system. See Delta
Pax3, Pax6	Paired box gene 3, Paired box gene 6
Pdgfra	Platelet-derived growth factor receptor A, a receptor on the surface of many cells
pErk	Phosphorylated ERK, a FGF8 effector
Prickle 1	Prickle homolog 1 protein is part of the noncanonical Wnt signaling pathway that helps regulate the polarized deposition of fibronectin on the surface of cells undergoing movements of convergence extension during gastrulation
RALDH2, Raldh2	Retinaldehyde dehydrogenase 2, an RA-synthesizing enzyme
RAREs	Retinoic acid response elements
RA	Retinoic acid, a major signaling molecule that establishes a longitudinal gradient across the developing embryo from higher levels cephalically to lower levels caudally. Strongly related to the Hox gene code and to the specific craniocaudal identity of each body segment
Rdh10	Retinol dehydrogenase 10, an RA-synthesizing enzyme, together with Radlh2
Ripply1, Ripply2	Genes that encode the nuclear protein transcriptional repressors ripply1 and ripply2 required for vertebrate somitogenesis. Mesp2 activates Ripply1 & 2 which eliminate the Tbx6 protein precisely over the length of the newly forming somite. The anterior edge of the newly displaced Tbx6 signal then specifies the anterior border of the next somite to form. In mice, absence leads to early postnatal death with a malsegmented axial skeleton
RXR-RARs	Retinoid X receptors (RXRs) heterodimerize with retinoic acid receptors (RARs) in order to bind to nuclear DNA

(continued on next page)

Table 1 (continued)	
Term	**Definition, Description, Action**
SNAI1	A zinc-finger protein encoded by the SNAI1 gene; part of a family of transcription factors that promote the repression of the E-cadherin adhesion molecule to regulate EMT
Sox1 and Sox2	SRY (sex determining region Y)-box 1 (and 2), transcription factors involved in maintaining embryonic stem cells and specifying neural fates
TBXT	*Brachyury* (previously *T* or *Bra*) is key to maintaining the neuromesodermal progenitor niche, by creating the high Wnt and low RA concentrations needed to maintain cells in a progenitor state
Tbx6	T-box transcription factor 6. Cells adopting a paraxial mesodermal fate upregulate Tbx6
Wnts	The wingless family of signaling proteins that initiate many of the systems in embryogenesis of the spine
Wnt3a	A key member of the Wnt family, notable for initiating expression of the Hox genes and for establishing gradients in the caudal spine

Abbreviations: CNS, central nervous system; EMT, epithelial-mesenchymal transition; EPHA4, Ephrin receptor A4; MESGN1, mesogenin 1; MESP, mesoderm posterior; RA, retinoic acid; RALDH2, retinaldehyde dehydrogenase 2; RARs, RA receptors; RAREs, RA response elements; SPRY2, sprouty 2; TBXT, transcription factor Brachyury; TCF15, transcription factor 15; TGF-β, transforming growth factor beta.
Auleha A, Pourquié O. Signaling gradients during paraxial mesoderm development. 2010. Cold Spring Harbor Perspect Biol 2010;2:a000869. https://doi.org/10.1101/cshperspet.a000869; Wikipedia, separately for each item.

often reinforce each other to establish a positive feedback loop that maintains and increases the concentrations of both signals. Alternatively, the molecular signals may antagonize each other to limit the signal available to specific cells or to restrict signaling to specific physical locations. The molecular signals may activate a system that produces a gene product that then inhibits its own production, until decreasing levels of that signal permit the system to reactivate. Such systems generate oscillations in signal intensity creating on, off, and on-again fluctuations in molecular signals and cell fate.

Two common systems for establishing gradients are the source-sink model and the messenger RNA (mRNA) decay model.

Source-sink model

In this system, active signal is produced at one point, diffuses outward from that point, and is actively degraded at a different point, establishing a decreasing concentration gradient from high (at synthesis site) to low (at degradation site). The gradient of retinoic acid (RA) is established in this way.[1]

Messenger RNA decay model (gradient by inheritance model; cell lineage transport model)

A signaling gradient may also be established by an mRNA decay mechanism, in which gene transcription produces intracellular mRNA only at a specific source. As those cells migrate away from the source and divide, the mRNA concentration within each daughter cell decreases progressively. Less mRNA means less gene product, so the decreasing mRNA gradient becomes translated into a decreasing gradient of the signaling molecule. At steady state, the remaining mRNA concentration and diminishing molecular signal then reflect the time since the cell left the zone of production. Gradients of fibroblast growth factor (FGF) and Wnt are produced this way.

Key Signaling Molecules/Systems

Fibroblast growth factors

FGFs are a family of polypeptide morphogens that serve mainly as secreted signaling molecules. They diffuse outward from their point of production, forming a diminishing concentration gradient that helps to specify cell fates in a dose-dependent manner.[2] Molecularly, the FGF morphogens are ligands that bind with a high degree of specificity to cell surface FGF receptor tyrosine kinases. In vertebrates, 4 highly related FGF receptors (FGFR1–FGFR4) and multiple isoforms of the receptors can bind the FGF ligands with variable degrees of specificity. FGF receptors consist of an extracellular ligand-binding domain, a transmembrane domain, and a cytoplasmic tyrosine kinase domain. Binding of the FGF ligand to the receptor causes dimerization of the FGF receptor and activation of tyrosine that then further directs downstream signal transduction pathways.[3] In the spine, a gradient of Fgf8 extends along the anteroposterior axis from low (cranial) to high (caudal). The gradient of Fgf strongly influences segmentation of the somites, including setting the level at which each new epithelial somite separates itself from the mesenchymal presomitic mesoderm.

In mice FGF3 is an essential factor for coordination of neural tube development with axis extension. FGF3 is secreted from the mesodermal layer, which drives axis extension, and negatively regulates expression of bone morphogenetic proteins (BMPs). In the absence of FGF3, excess BMP (1) negatively affects the mesoderm, causing premature termination of the embryologic axis; and (2) stimulates the neuroepithelium causing neuroepithelial proliferation, delay in neural tube closure, and premature specification of neural crest.[4]

Wnts/β-catenin

The Wnts are a key gene family of secreted glycolipoproteins named for their homology to 2 *Drosophila* genes: *wg* (wingless) and *int-1* (first proto-oncogene functioning to integrate elements into the genome).[5] There are 19 Wnt genes in most mammalian genomes. β-Catenin is a cytoplasmic protein that in humans is encoded by the *CTNNB1* gene. In the absence of Wnt signaling, β-catenin is produced and degraded within the cytoplasm, keeping its cytoplasmic concentration low. In a highly complex cascade, Wnt signaling acts to prevent the degradation of β-catenin, allowing its levels to increase in the cytoplasm. High cytoplasmic levels of β-catenin enable β-catenin to enter the nucleus, where it acts to derepress Wnt target genes. This complex, multistep process involves binding of Wnt to the 7-pass-transmembrane receptor Frizzled and to its coreceptor the low-density lipoprotein receptor–related protein 6 (LRP6) (or LRP5), alterations in the scaffolding proteins Dishevelled (Dvl) and axin, and a further signaling cascade. Noncanonical Wnt signaling pathways also exist. Wnt signaling was reviewed by MacDonald and colleagues[6] in 2009 and Gao and colleagues[7] in 2014.

Wnt3 is essential for the formation of the primitive streak; for gastrulation; for initiating transcription of the homeobox (Hox) genes; for maintaining the neuromesodermal stem cell progenitor niche; for directing progenitors toward a mesodermal, not neural, fate; and, by all these measures, for forming the spine caudal to the occipital somites.[8] Stem cells exposed to signaling by both FGFs and Wnts begin to express key transcription factors such as CDX1, CDX2, and CDX4; Brachyury (formerly T/Bra; now transcription factor Brachyury [TBXT]); and SOX2, and go on to differentiate into spinal cord progenitors that express cervical and thoracic Hox genes.[9] Wnt3 mutant embryos do not express any Hox genes and generate neural progenitor cells whose caudal limit is the hindbrain and cervical spinal cord.[9] The signal inherent to posteriorization of the body axis in bilaterians is the Wnt-dependent stabilization of β-catenin. This functions as a master regulator to initiate Hox gene expression at a suitable time point in the embryo.[8]

Brachyury

Brachyury (previously T or Bra, now TBXT) is the key regulator of the molecular signaling environment of the neuromesodermal progenitor niche. Brachyury creates the environment of high Wnt and low RA concentration needed to maintain cells in a progenitor state. In mice and humans, TBXT directly activates Wnt ligand transcription. In turn, Wnt signaling upregulates TBXT expression, creating a positive autoregulatory loop that maintains high Wnt levels in the progenitor zone. TBXT also directly activates transcription of the enzyme cytochrome p450 26a1 (cyp26a1), which degrades RA, so brachyury also maintains the low level of RA in the progenitor zone. Brachyury is required to complete posterior axis extension.

Retinoic acid

All-trans-RA is synthesized in the body stepwise from all-trans-retinol to retinaldehyde to all-trans-RA. RA is synthesized in the anterior presomitic mesoderm and somites of the developing spine by the RA biosynthetic enzyme retinaldehyde dehydrogenase 2 (RALDH2). RA is then degraded more posteriorly in the neuromesodermal progenitor stem cell niche by the RA-degrading enzyme cyp26a1. This system establishes and maintains a gradient of RA that diminishes from anterior to posterior. The low posterior level of RA is required to maintain the integrity of the stem cell niche for neuromesodermal precursors at the caudal end of the developing embryo. Functional RA response elements have been identified in the regions flanking the 3′ end of several Hox genes.

Because the gradient of RA signaling is highly correlated with the Hox code, mutations or exogenous factors that alter the concentration of RA may influence the Hox code to respecify segment identity, as, say, C6 or T1 instead of C7. Alterations in RA concentration are also associated with severe cardiac and vascular malformations.[10] The increased RA signaling decreases endothelial cell proliferation, leading to premature coalescence and differentiation of precursors, and impaired vascular remodeling later on.[10] Increased concentration of RA in the neuromesodermal progenitor niche, whether by increased production or reduced degradation, may cause the extensive anorectal, urogenital, spinal, and lower extremity disorder of sirenomelia.

Bone morphogenetic protein

BMPs and the related growth and differentiation factors are members of the transforming growth factor β (TGF-β) family. They transduce their signals through type I and type II serine-threonine kinase receptors and their intracellular downstream effectors, including the Smad proteins.[11] BMP signaling plays a major role in primary neurulation and interacts with other signaling gradients, such as FGF and RA, to coordinate primary neurulation with secondary neurulation and axis extension. The levels of BMP, RA, and FGF influence both the neural and the mesodermal cell population. Increased levels of BMP increase proliferation of the neuroepithelium, delay neural tube closure, and cause premature specification of neural crest.[4] After neural tube closure, BMP4 signaling is required for delaminating of the neural crest.[4] Increased levels of BMP also deplete progenitors from the presomitic mesoderm and may lead to premature termination of axis elongation.[4] This effect may be countered by FGF and RA. FGF3 derived from the caudal presomitic mesoderm regulates BMP signals in the adjacent neuroepithelium. Mice lacking Fgf3 show premature axis termination.[4] RA decreases BMP signal duration by reducing the level of phosphorylated Smad1, an intracellular component of the BMP signaling pathway.[10]

Access to chromosomes

Along their length, chromosomes are partitioned into large segments called topologically associating domains (TADs) and subdomains (subTADs) (Fig. 1).[12] These domains help determine a regulatory landscape that restricts regulatory input to the genes in time and space. The cis-regulatory landscape consists of enhancers, insulators, and other architectural elements that can be located proximal to the gene or dispersed over large genomic distances. The trans-factor modifications consist of posttranscriptional modifications to the gene product. Together, these systems regulate expression of multiple systems, notably the Hox code for specifying the specific identify of each segment along the anterior-posterior axis of the body.

The chromosome containing the HoxA gene has 3 topological zones: a 3′ subTAD, a middle subTAD situated 5′ to the early HoxA genes, and a distal 5′ segment that contains Hoxa13 and its associated enhancers (see Fig. 1).[12] The chromatin conformation of the 3′ subTAD is open for early Wnt activation. The middle subTAD harbors cis elements that are initially fully covered by repressive histone modifications and that require Cdx-driven chromatin modification to allow access to the DNA. Because the Wnts also induce the expression of the Cdx genes, the Cdx transcription factors serve as secondary activators to open the mid-Hox genes for transcription. The 5′ TAD does not contain early Wnt-responsive enhancers. This subTAD compartmentalization of the HoxA cluster and its flanking regulatory domains seems to underlie the segmental, and relatively independent, activation of the anterior versus posterior genes of each Hox cluster.

Hox code

During development, the Hox genes specify the positional identity of each segment along the anteroposterior axis of the body. The homeotic genes are situated on 4 separate chromosomes in 4 separate clusters, each containing a subset of 13 evolutionarily conserved genes. The 4 clusters, designated HoxA to HoxD, seem to represent duplication and reduplication of an originally single set of homeotic genes, giving rise to 4 paralogous gene clusters on the 4 different chromosomes. Within each cluster, the Hox genes are arrayed along the chromosome in order from the 3′ to the 5′ end of the chromosome; for example, Hoxa1 (at the 3′ end) through Hoxa13 (at the 5′ end) of the same chromosome.

Each set of Hox genes shows colinearity. Within each cluster, the Hox genes are activated in the same order from 1 to 13 as the order in which they are (1) expressed during embryogenesis (temporal colinearity) and in which (2) they specify the identity of each body segment from cranial to caudal (spatial colinearity). As the embryo lengthens, the sequential activation of Hox genes over time provides the precursors of embryonic tissues with position-specific Hox information along the trunk axis. Notably, Wnt3a initiates the activation of the first, most 3′ gene of each Hox cluster.

Two Hox-Hox interactions are important[13–15]:

Posterior induction. Expression of each anterior Hox gene induces the expression of the more posterior Hox genes. This induction of sequentially more posterior genes drives Hox temporal colinearity and the sequential anteroposterior expression of each gene in the cluster.

Posterior prevalence. Within each cluster, expression of each Hox gene represses the expression of the Hox genes anterior to it. Because the Hox code helps determine the anterior-posterior identity of each segment, posterior prevalence translates the sequential temporal pattern of expression into a set of signals that specify progressively more posterior segment identity. Posterior prevalence converts temporal

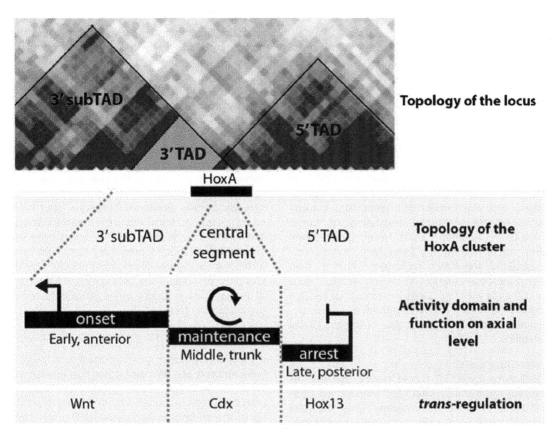

Fig. 1. Cis-regulatory and trans-regulatory features of the HoxA locus from initiation of transcription to the completion of axis elongation. (*Top*) On the chromosome, the HoxA locus lies between the 3′ TAD and the 5′ TAD, in relation to a proximally situated 3′ subTAD. (*Bottom*) The HoxA cluster and its flanking regions may be partitioned into 3 functional segments: the 3′ subTAD, a central portion, and the 5′ TAD. The 3′ subTAD is activated early by Wnt signals in the induction domain of the anterior-most HoxA genes. Following initial Wnt-mediated induction of 3′ HoxA genes, the central part of the HoxA cluster is activated by Cdx transcription factors. Cdx activation of the gene ensures that central Hox genes are expressed to maintain the axial progenitors of the trunk and to pattern trunk tissues. The 5′ portion of HoxA contains and regulates Hoxa13, which is expressed late and is responsible for the arrest of axial elongation. (*From* Neijts R, Deschamps J. At the base of colinear Hox gene expression: cis-features and trans-factors orchestrating the initial phase of Hox cluster activation. Developmental Biology 2017;428:293–299. p. 297; with permission.)

colinearity into spatial colinearity. For this reason, delay in expression of any 1 of the Hox genes is tantamount to loss of that gene's function, altering segment identity and position. The Hox clusters are highly responsive to exogenous RA signals from early stages onward, so the gradients of RA help establish the colinear Hox expression in human pluripotent cells. However, a role for endogenous RA in initial Hox induction in vertebrates remains to be established.[12]

Cdx genes

The caudal-like homeobox genes, Cdx1, Cdx2, and Cdx4, function to provide access to the chromosome for transcription of the midrange (trunk segment) of the 13 Hox genes. Cdx and Hox genes both derive from an ancient protoHox gene or gene cluster and both are induced by Wnt signals. Along the 3′ portions of the HoxA and HoxB gene clusters, the chromatin is open and the DNA is available for gene transcription. Cdx genes are not required for the initial activation of the 3′ Hox genes. However, within the middle (trunk) portion of the Hox clusters, Cdx is required at several cis-regulatory elements to alter the chromatin landscape and make the DNA accessible.[12,13,16] During progressive colinear Hox expression, the Cdx-activated Hox genes shift from a covered inactive chromatin domain to an open active domain and may loop out of their chromosome territory to expose the genes for transcription. Cdx genes are required for axial extension of the body. All 3 Cdx genes contribute to this function, the most potent being Cdx2. Total absence of Cdx genes leads to total absence of the body posterior to the occipital somites.

Delta-Notch lateral inhibition

Delta-Notch signaling is a dominance-submission interaction between 2 adjacent cells in which (1) ligands on the surface of the signal-sending (dominant) cell bind to (2) Notch receptors on the surface of the receiving (sub-missive) cell.[17] By a complex cascade, this releases a second signal from the receiving cell membrane, which then translocates to the nucleus, where it interacts with the CSL transcription factor complex (short for *CBF1* in humans, *Suppressor of Hairless* in *Drosophila*, *Lag-1* in *Caenorhabditis elegans*), thereby achieving transcriptional regulation of target genes. In addition, Delta-Notch interactions may occur within the same cell, functionally neutralizing the Notch receptors within its own cell (a process designated cis inhibition).[17] As a result, cells with high Delta levels cannot receive signals via Notch, converting them into unidirectional signal-sending cells during lateral inhibition.

Oscillating genes

Oscillating (cyclic or clock) genes use autorepressor gene transcription factors to create oscillations in gene expression. They typically encode basic loop-helix-loop (bHLH) transcription factors, such as Hairy1, Hairy2, and Lunatic fringe (Lfng) (in chick); hairy and enhancer of split 1 (Hes1), Hes7, and Lfng (in mouse); and Hairy and enhancer of spilt-related 1 (Her1) and Her7 in zebrafish.[18,19] The continuous on-and-off switching of gene expression gives rise to oscillations. The oscillations of these cyclic genes establish the somitogenesis clock. The time delay from gene transcription to protein translation to protein degradation and subsequent reactivation of the gene sets the period of the segmentation clock. Vertebrates seem to use the conserved autorepressor loop from the *hairy* and *Enhancer of split* gene family as the core oscillators.[19] Such a mechanism requires that the half-lives of the mRNA and the protein both need to be very short to allow rapid oscillation.[13]

ESTABLISHMENT OF THE AXIS
Initial Allocation of Tissue

The traditional view of spinal embryogenesis is that future neural cells are initially induced with anterior (forebrain) identity and that caudalizing signals then convert a portion of these to a posterior spinal fate. This initial activation and later transformation model is now challenged. Current work[9] suggests, instead, that there is an early developmental time window during which epiblast cells are preconfigured for neural induction that commits them to a regional (anterior vs posterior) identity before they acquire specific neural identity.[9] That is, embryonic stem cells first acquire a regional, axial identity before they acquire a specifically neural identity (**Fig. 2**). One mechanism for this may be stage-specific remodeling of the chromatin by the Cdx transforming factors. This mechanism would limit access to genetic signals, creating a major anterior-posterior division in the nervous system between the spinal cord and the more rostral territories.[9] In vertebrates, the anterior nervous system (forebrain, midbrain, and hindbrain) are formed from cells in the anterior epiblast. The more caudal somites and spinal cord are formed from bipotent progenitor cells that arise within the caudal lateral epiblast (tailbud). This dichotomy may reflect the persistence in bilaterians of the earlier organization of the nervous system in the cnidarians (see **Fig. 2**).

Specification of Axial (Craniocaudal) Identify

In the mouse embryo, gastrulation starts in the posterior epiblast, at a site demarcated by expression of Wnt3 and Brachyury.[12] During early gastrulation the primitive streak gradually extends toward the distal tip of the embryonic egg cylinder. The first Hox-positive region in the embryo is the very posterior part of the fully extended primitive streak (**Fig. 3**). After the 3′-most Hox gene is turned on in the posterior streak area, its expression domain spreads anteriorly (ie, cephalically) by a process that does not involve cell migration. The transcript domain then reaches the anterior part of the primitive streak where the node streak domain lies within the anterior streak just caudal to the node, and where the paired, flanking caudal lateral epiblastic zones maintain axial progenitor cells, including bipotent neuromesodermal progenitor cells.

After initial activation of the 3′ (anterior) Hox genes, progressively more 5′ (posterior) Hox genes begin to be transcribed in the posterior streak area. As with the earlier genes, the expression domains of the later genes also spread anteriorly. Sequentially therefore, the progenitor cells within the anterior node streak domain and caudal lateral epiblast express progressively more and more posterior Hox genes (**Figs. 4** and **5**). The precise timing of early Hox initiation in the primitive streak is a first and determinant step for the later organization of the Hox expression boundaries in the embryo.[12]

AXIS ELONGATION

After the end of gastrulation, new presomitic mesodermal cells arise within a progenitor (stem cell) niche in the tailbud.[13]

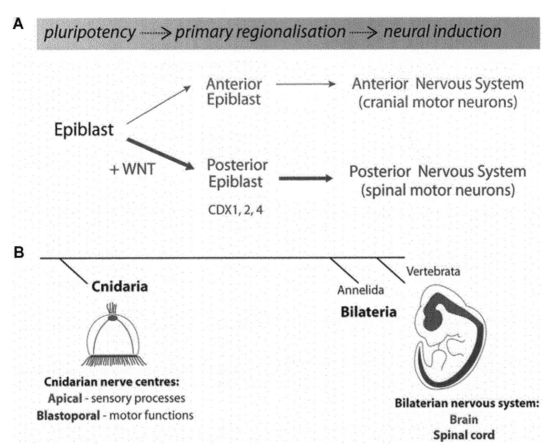

Fig. 2. Proposed model of nervous system development. (A) Early in embryogenesis, molecular signaling directs pluripotent epiblast cells to either anterior (*blue*) or posterior (*red*) cell populations before the cells acquire specific neural identity. Anteriorized epiblast cells ultimately generate the anterior nervous system; posteriorized epiblast cells generate the spinal cord. (B) Cnidarians display 2 distinct nerve centers: an apical center (*blue*) and a blastoporal center (*red*), which express putative CDX orthologs. Comparisons between cnidarian and bilaterian animals suggest that the present anterior-posterior organization of vertebrate central nervous systems may have arisen through expansion and merging of the 2 distinct nerve centers already present in cnidarians. (*From* Metzis V. et al. Nervous system regionalization entails axial allocation before neural differentiation. Cell 2018;175(Nov. 1):1105–1118. p. 1115; with permission.)

Progenitor Niche

Overall, the anteroposterior elongation of the embryo involves cell proliferation within the maintained posterior stem cell niches, specification of these initially bipotent cells to be future mesoderm or neural tissue, migration of the modified progenitor cells into separate transitional maturation zones, and subsequent migration of the newly specified cells out of those zones into proper position to form the mesodermal somites and spinal cord. In actuality, maturation and specification of progenitor cells is far more complex and shows significant species variability.[20–24]

Following gastrulation, a stem cell population of bipotent neuromesodermal progenitor cells persists in the stem cell niche between the node and the cranial end of the neural groove (Figs. 6 and 7). In diverse species, this zone is designated variably as the node streak border, caudolateral epiblast, caudoneural hinge, or tailbud.[22] The stem cell character of this niche is maintained by a specific molecular signaling environment of high Wnt and low RA levels. The levels of Wnt and RA interact in positive feedback loops to maintain the niche. Within the niche, the neuromesodermal progenitors are characterized by a specific pattern (signature) of molecular expression, including the mesoderm-inducing TBXT, and the epiblast and neural transcription factors Sox2, Sox3, and Nkx1-2.[21,22] Neuromesodermal stem cells generate neural and paraxial presomitic mesoderm cells, which are the progenitors of the spinal cord and musculoskeleton of the trunk and tail respectively.

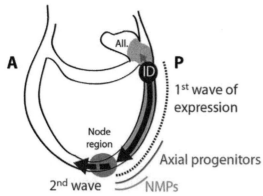

Fig. 3. Two early waves of Hox expression in the posterior of the embryo. At this stage, the embryo is folded into a faintly U shape, so the posterior end of the embryo (P) lies behind, not yet caudal to, the anterior end (A) (see **Fig. 4**). Wave 1: Hoxa1 expression (*purple*) initiates in the most posterior end of the primitive streak at the induction domain (ID). From the induction domain, the earliest Hox-expressing cells pass outward (*small arrow*) to contribute to extraembryonic tissue (the allantois [all]). Thereafter, Hoxa expression spreads anteriorly (*large purple arrow*) toward the anterior end of the primitive streak and the node region, which harbor axial progenitor cells, including neuromesodermal progenitors (NMPs). Thereafter, in sequence, cells expressing progressively more posterior Hox genes repeat the same entry and anterior-spreading expression dynamics, also reaching the node region. As a consequence, over time, the neuromesodermal progenitors sequentially express more and more posterior Hox genes. Wave 2: the Hox expression acquired by the axial progenitors in the node region is transmitted to the descendants of these progenitors, and regulated independently, to form future neuroectoderm and mesoderm, contributing to the elongating axis. The primitive streak is indicated by a dashed line. (*From* Neijts R, Deschamps J. At the base of colinear Hox gene expression: cis-features and trans-factors orchestrating the initial phase of Hox cluster activation. Developmental Biology 2017;428:293–299. p. 294; with permission.)

Further Maturation

Signaling systems direct the bipotential neuromesodermal progenitor cells toward either mesodermal or neural fates (see **Figs. 6** and **7**). At present, it is thought that mutual repression between paraxial mesoderm transcription programs and neural transcription programs generates a "toggle switch" that causes the neuromesodermal progenitor cells to adopt either a mesodermal or a neural identity. However, at least some of these progenitor cells have been found to contribute progeny to both future mesoderm and future neural fates.

Toward presomitic mesoderm: Wnt3a, Mesogenin1, and Tbx6

Wnt3a induces the bipotential neuromesodermal cells to become mesodermal, not neural, progenitors by activating Mesogenin1 (*Msgn1*) a master regulator of presomitic mesodermal differentiation. *Msgn1* directs the neuromesodermal progenitors to a presomitic (and later somitic) mesodermal state by activating *Tbx6, Snai1 Foxc1, Pdgfra*, and *Dact1*, all of which are essential for mesodermal development. In addition, Msgn1 inhibits cell entry into a neural fate by directly activating the transcription factor *Tbx6*, a known inhibitor of the neural determinant *Sox2*. *Tbx6* suppresses *Sox2*, and thereby suppresses neural fates. Suppression of Sox2 seems to be required for mesodermal differentiation, because embryos lacking *Tbx6* form ectopic neural tissue in place of somites. Further, forced expression of Sox2 in caudal paraxial mesoderm converts presumptive mesoderm into neural tissue, and misexpression of Sox2 in paraxial mesoderm is sufficient to generate ectopic neural tubes.[21] Notably, *Msgn1* is expressed only in the mesenchymal cells of the presomitic mesoderm and only at the time of their maturation, making Msgn1 a tissue-specific and stage-specific transcription factor.[21]

Toward preneural states and the spinal cord

Data suggest that cells en route from the epiblast to the spinal cord transition through at least 3 distinct transcriptional stages: neuromesodermal progenitor, preneural progenitor, and neural progenitor.

Preneural tube Cells exiting the neuromesodermal progenitor niche to a neural fate remain in the epiblastic layer of the embryo and enter a transition zone in the caudal neural plate designated the preneural tube (pre-NT). This transition zone lies between the tail of the embryo that harbors neuromesodermal progenitors and the neural progenitors of the spinal cord. The pre-NT cells are morphologically and molecularly distinct from both the early neuromesodermal progenitors and the later neural progenitors of the spinal cord. They form a well-ordered, pseudostratified epithelium that begins to undergo the morphogenetic movements involved in neural tube closure. They no longer express the TBXT found in neuromesodermal progenitors, but, unlike neural progenitors in the spinal cord, they do express Nkx1-2. Fgf signaling remains active in the pre-NT and maintains the pre-NT state by promoting proliferation and by blocking the expression of *Pax6, Irx3*, and other transcription factors characteristic of neural progenitors.

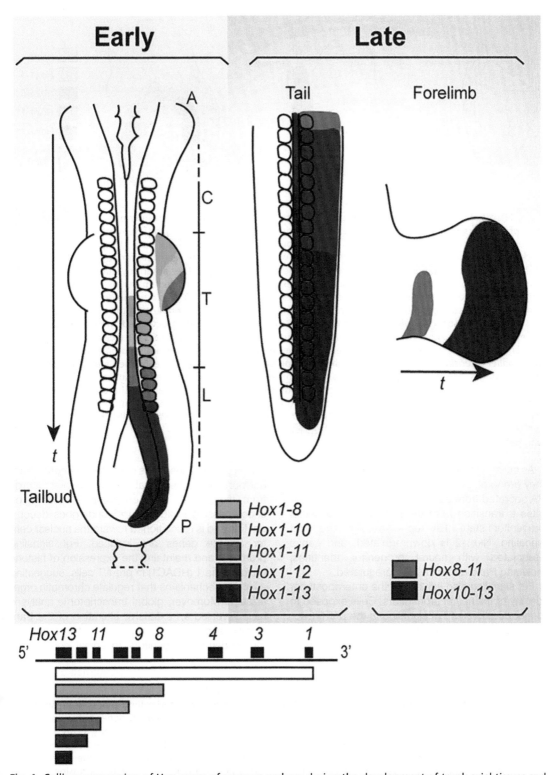

Fig. 4. Collinear expression of Hox genes of a mouse embryo during the development of trunk axial tissues and limbs. In the schema of the chromosome (*bottom*), the 3′ end is shown to the reader's right and the 5′ end to the reader's left. Early: posteriorly overlapping transcript domains of HoxD genes in the developing neural tube (*midline*); somites of the cervical (C), thoracic (T), and lumbar (L) regions; forelimb mesoderm (lateral bulges), and nascent mesoderm and neuroectoderm in the tailbud. Note the spatial and temporal collinearity.

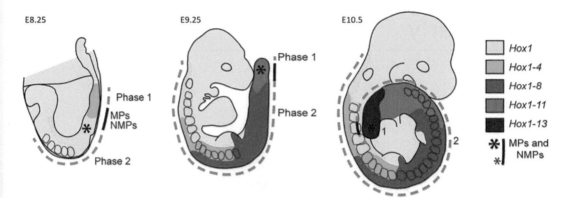

Fig. 5. Phases of maturation. Phase 1: the early temporal colinearity of Hox gene transcription is translated by the axial progenitors into spatially colinear expression domains in the emerging differentiated tissues. E8.25. In sequence, the transcript domains of Hox1 followed by Hox2, Hox3, and Hox4 (phase 1) expand anteriorly and reach the axial progenitor region (*large asterisk*) that will become the stem cell niche for neuromesodermal progenitors (NMPs) and mesodermal progenitors (MPs) before expanding further anteriorly during phase 2 (spatial colinearity). E9.25. Transcriptional initiation of the next Hox genes has occurred (midtrunk Hox4 to Hox8), and activation of more posterior Hox genes takes place (as shown with Hox11). The expression domains expand anteriorly toward the axial progenitor area in those tissues generated by the descendants of the mesodermal progenitors and neuromesodermal progenitors. E10.5. Hox13 is now transcriptionally activated and expressed strongly posteriorly, where it counteracts further axial extension. The Wnt and Fgf pathways are weakened, and the progenitor niche becomes deficient, with fewer and fewer mesoderm progenitors and neuromesodermal progenitors (*smaller asterisk*). The color code identifies the combinations of Hox genes expressed along the axis at the different stages. Mesodermal progenitors and neuromesodermal progenitors are found around the anterior part of the primitive streak, just posterior to the node (indentation) at E8.25 and in the tailbud at E9.25 and E10.5. Because the embryo turns, anterior is to the left for the E8.25 embryo but toward the top for the E9.25 and E10.5 embryos. (*From* Deschamps J, Duboule D. Embryonic timing, axial stem cells, chromatin dynamics, and the Hox clock. Genes & Development 2017;31:1406–1416. https://doi.org/10.1101/gad.303123.117, p 1409; with permission.)

As cells exit the pre-NT and enter the spinal cord they are exposed to increasing concentrations of RA secreted from adjacent somites. This precipitates a transition from the preneural to a neural progenitor state. RA represses Fgf and Wnt signaling. Nkx1-2 is downregulated, and genes associated with neural progenitor identities, including Pax6 and Irx3, are upregulated.

Fgf signaling also influences the anteroposterior identity of the neural progenitors. Cells exposed to longer durations of Fgf signaling in the pre-NT acquire progressively more posterior fates, as shown by their temporal induction of progressively more

5′ Hox genes. These cells contribute to more posterior portions of the spinal cord when they emerge from the pre-NT. The chromatin in the region encompassing Pax6 and Irx3 undergoes decompaction and is repositioned toward the nuclear center as the genes are induced. Fgf signaling promotes and maintains the expression of histone deacetylase 1 (HDAC1) in pre-NT cells, suggesting a link to mechanisms that regulate chromatin organization. Moreover, global transcriptome analyses have revealed an extensive alteration of the transcriptional program during the transition from neuromesodermal progenitors to spinal cord neural

---

Hox1 is expressed from an anterior limit that is the most rostral of all Hox genes in the embryo (expression not shown in the embryo; no color in the bar), and Hox8 is expressed from an anterior limit that is less rostral than that of Hox1 in the embryo. Posterior to this Hox8 anterior expression boundary, all genes between 1 and 8 are expressed (green color in the embryo and in the bar corresponding with Hox8). Similarly, posterior to the Hox10 expression boundary in the embryo, all genes between Hox1 and Hox10 are expressed (lighter blue in the embryo and in the bar corresponding with Hox10), and similar representations illustrate the expression of Hox11, Hox12, and Hox13. These domains thus tend to overlap posteriorly in the embryo. Expression of other Hox genes is not shown. Late: Hox transcript distribution in the developing tailbud and forelimb bud. Color codes indicate the cumulative combinations of Hox transcripts. Anterior is to the top in all schemes. A, anterior; P, posterior; t, time of anterior to posterior development (*From* Deschamps J, Duboule D. Embryonic timing, axial stem cells, chromatin dynamics, and the Hox clock. Genes & Development 2017;31:1406–1416. pg. 1407; with permission.)

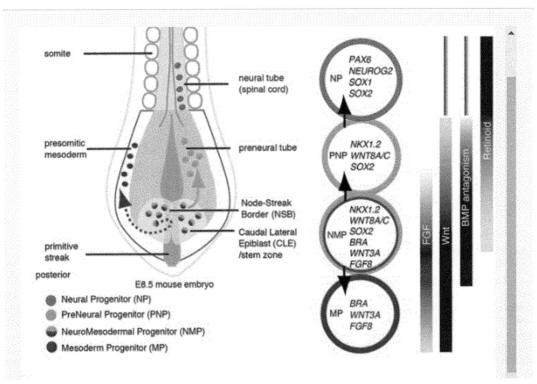

Fig. 6. Factors influencing the maturation of the neuromesodermal progenitor like cells into both neural and mesodermal structures. The mouse E8.5 caudal embryo with color coding of cell types and related signaling molecules (*circles*). The opposing signaling gradients of FGF, Wnts, BMP, and retinoids signal bipotential NMPs to migrate outward from the progenitor niche within the caudal lateral epiblast and differentiate along 2 lines. Cells differentiating along the mesodermal line form mesodermal progenitors within the presomitic mesoderm and mature into mesodermal progenitors (MP) within the developing somites. Cells differentiating along the neural line form preneural progenitors (PNP) within a preneural tube and mature into neural progenitors (NP) within the developing neural tube. Bra is an old abbreviation for brachyury. Gradient directionality is displayed vertically on the right. (*From* Verrier L. et al. Neural differentiation, selection and transcriptomic profiling of human neuromesodermal progenitor-like cells in vitro. Development 2018; 145(16):dev 166215. p. 16; with permission.)

progenitor. These alterations include changes in the cell cycle, RNA processing, and protein degradation machineries. Thus substantial changes in the chromatin structure and the transcriptome occur during the differentiation of neuromesodermal progenitors to preneural tube and neural progenitors.

Primary neural tube Fate mapping studies in the chick show that all of the material forming the caudal neural tube below the upper thoracic level is generated precociously in the transient node streak border[22,23] (see Jena L. Miller and Thierry A.G.M. Huisman's article, "Spinal Dysraphia, Chiari 2 Malformation, Unified Theory and Advances in Fetoscopic Repair," in this issue).

NORMAL SOMITOGENESIS

The segmented body axis is established by a process of somitogenesis, in which the paired unsegmented columns of presomitic mesoderm are periodically and progressively divided into bilaterally symmetric epithelial somites. As in a production line, where raw material enters at one end and finished product emerges at the other, progenitor mesodermal cells enter the caudal end of the pipeline, undergo transformation, and emerge at the cephalic end of the pipeline as newly formed somites. Rhythmically and repeatedly, the entire process proceeds progressively more posteriorly, making somite after somite, until axis elongation is complete.

Somitic Clock

During somitogenesis, the presomitic mesoderm can be divided into 2 major functional regions (**Figs. 8** and **9**).[13] At the caudal end of the presomitic mesoderm, the individual cells show an intrinsic oscillatory expression of transcription

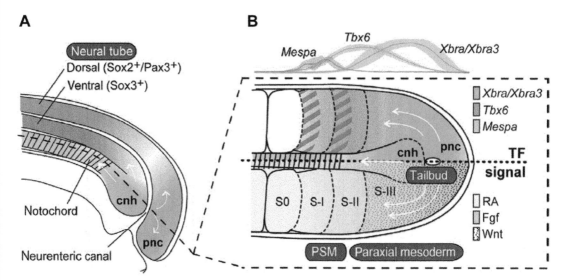

Fig. 7. (*A*, *B*) A possible T-box factor-dependent genetic regulatory network for specifying neuromesodermal trajectories within the terminal growth zone of *Xenopus* embryo at early tailbud stage. Sagittal (*A*) and horizontal (*B*) sections through the posterior region of an early tailbud embryo illustrate the patterns of expression of Xbra/Xbra3, Tbx6, Mespa, Sox2/3, and Pax3; the signaling activity of FGF, Wnt, and RA; and the recruitment of mesodermal and neural cells (*white arrows*) from the chordoneural hinge (cnh) and posterior wall of the neurenteric canal (pnc). Most cells of the cnh give rise to the notochord and the ventrolateral horns of the neural tube, whereas cells in the pnc contribute to paraxial mesoderm and the dorsal roof of the neural tube. S0 is newly forming somite; S-I, S-II, and S-III are presomitic mesoderm (PSM). The graph above (*B*) shows semiquantitative measurements of transcript levels within the tailbud. (*From* Gentsch GE et al. Chapter 5. Cooperation between T-box factors regulates the continuous segregation of germ layers during vertebrate embryogenesis. Curr Topics Dev Biology 2017;122:117–159, Fig. 5, page 137; with permission.)

factors, under the control of clock genes. The period of their oscillations is the somitic clock. These genes are under control of both the gradients of FGF, Wnt, and Notch and the differing oscillation frequencies of the Wnt and Notch signals, among others. Initially, the oscillation frequencies of the individual presomitic cells are "noisy" and unsynchronized. Rhythmically and repeatedly, over each clock period: (1) the oscillations of the individual cells become entrained and synchronized; (2) the now-synchronous cell oscillations interact with the preexisting gradients and oscillations of FGF, Wnt, and Notch signals; and (3) by an unresolved mechanism, at a specific signal, these interactions lead to sudden, near-simultaneous cessation of the intrinsic oscillations of the presomitic cells. The level at which oscillations cease is designated the determination front. Cephalic to the determination front, the developing cells begin to undergo mesenchymal-to-epithelial transition (MET), acquire the character of epithelial cells, and become the next newly formed somite. Caudal to the determination front, 1 level more posterior, the entire process repeats to produce the next somite. In humans, a new pair of somites forms about every 4 to 6 hours, to a total of 42–44 somites.[13] In the normal state, the left-sided and right-sided somites are generated with identical timing and spacing to form symmetric pairs.

Role of Delta-Notch Cell-Cell Interaction

During the clock period, the oscillations of the individual cells become entrained (synchronized) by cell migration, by Delta-Notch signaling between cells, and by induced periodic mitoses. The entering presomitic mesodermal progenitor cells incur multiple cell-cell contacts. During these contacts, Delta-Notch signaling between the cells entrains their individual oscillations to establish synchronous oscillations within the zone (discussed earlier in relation to key signaling molecules/systems and Delta-Notch lateral inhibition).[25] In addition, before entry into the presomitic mesoderm, the bipotential neuromesodermal progenitors are mostly held in the G2 stage of the cell cycle with few mitotic events. As these cells enter the mesodermal progenitor pool, they turn on *cdc25a*, a factor that promotes entry into mitosis. The concerted expression of cdc25a in cells entering the presomitic mesoderm causes synchronous mitoses, leading to doubling of the number of cells in the cell population. Because the 2

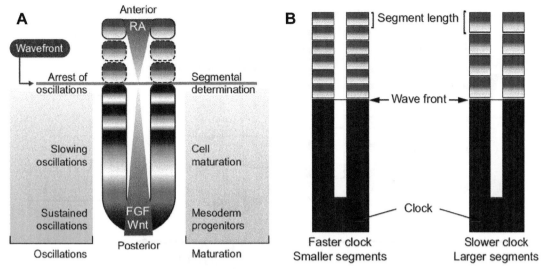

Fig. 8. Somitogenesis. (*A*) Global gradients control slowing and arrest of oscillating cells. An elongating vertebrate axis showing cyclic gene expression patterns in blue/white, arrested segments (*red/white with dashed boundaries*) and somites (*red/white with solid boundaries*). Gradients of FGF and Wnt (*brown*) span the tissue from the posterior. An opposing shorter-range gradient of RA (*gray*) expands caudally from the recently formed somites. The shape of these gradients is not known. Sustained high-frequency oscillations are observed in the posterior region of the tissue. Oscillators gradually slow down as they approach the wave front of arrest (the determination front) (*horizontal line*). (*Left*) The different stages that single-cell oscillators undergo as they traverse the tissue. (*Right*) The maturation program of presomitic mesoderm cells, running in parallel to segment length specification controlled by the clock. (*B*) The clock and wave front mechanism. Speed and numbers. The clock is created by oscillating gene expression in the presomitic mesoderm (*blue*). The wave front is created by a posteriorly moving front that arrests the oscillations of the clock. The resulting segments (*red/white*) have a length that is determined by the period of the clock multiplied by the regression velocity of the wave front. (*From* Oates AC, et al. Patterning embryos with oscillations: structure, function and dynamics of the vertebrate segmentation clock. Development 2012;139:625–639; with permission.)

daughter cells from each mitosis share the molecular components of the oscillator, they emerge into the pool with highly entrained clock oscillations, increasing the overall synchrony within the cell population. The essential function of Delta-Notch signaling in somite segmentation may be to establish and maintain synchrony of cell oscillation. In mammals, 2 notch and 2 delta are required for somitogenesis, which implies that 1 cyclic delta plus 1 noncyclic delta might be essential for securing the robustness of the synchronization.[19]

Determination Front

The molecular mechanisms by which the periodicity of the oscillations is regulated are not well understood.[18] Two major, likely interactive, mechanisms have been proposed to explain the determination front: gradient levels of signaling molecules, and differences in oscillation frequency. (1) Gradient levels. Presomitic mesoderm is patterned by the anterior to posterior gradient of RA opposing the caudal to cranial gradients of FGF and Wnts. As the body axis elongates posteriorly, these gradients

also shift posteriorly. As a result, the presomitic mesodermal cells that are situated at 1 specific point along the body axis experience a progressively more forward (ie, cephalic) level of these concentration gradients. The specific levels of these multiple gradients may establish the determination front.[26] (2) Differences in oscillation frequency. Many components of the Wnt, FGF, and Notch signaling pathway also oscillate. In mouse, the oscillations of the FGF8 effector pErk are thought to determine the pace of somitogenesis. The oscillation frequency of pErk varies little across the entire presomitic mesoderm. The oscillation frequency of Notch does vary along the presomitic mesoderm – developing somite. Caudally, the 2 frequencies are similar.[27] Toward the cephalic end of the future somite, Notch oscillations slow down, so the frequencies of the 2 oscillations become divergent. The difference in the 2 frequencies, and the consequent difference in the phases of their cycles, may mark the determination front. That is, the somite boundary may form where the wave of Notch expression is high and pErk expression is low.[26] However, carefully considered alternate interpretations of experimental data are offered by Wahi and

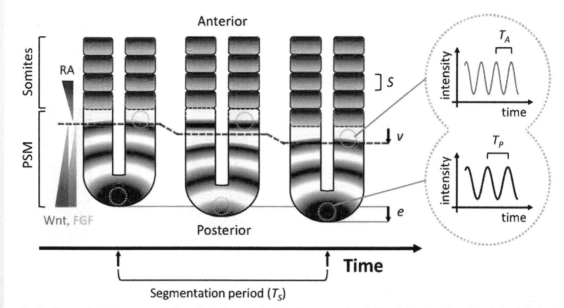

Fig. 9. The vertebrate segmentation clock. In vertebrates, the wave front (the determination front) (*red dashed line*) is influenced by Fgf and Wnt signaling gradients from the posterior end and a countergradient of RA arising from the somites further anteriorly. As the new somite forms and the axis elongates, the wave front sweeps posteriorly in concert. When the cyclic expression waves of *hes/her* genes (the blue color in the PSM) moves across the wave front, the oscillation arrests and a new segment boundary is determined. The frequencies of oscillation of multiple signaling molecules vary along the craniocaudal extent of the presomitic mesoderm and nascent somites. Blue or black dotted boxes represent nascent somites. (*From* Liao B-K, Oates AC. Delta-Notch signaling in segmentation. Arthropod Structure & Development 2017;46:432; with permission.)

colleagues[13] (2016) and Sonnen and colleagues[28] (2018), among others.

Somite Boundary Formation

Cephalic to the determination front, a genetic cascade leads to activation of mesoderm posterior 2 (Mesp2) by Notch in a Tbx6-dependent manner.[18] Behind the determination front, Mesp2 expression is inhibited by FGF activity, so the posterior cells remain as presomitic mesoderm. Starting immediately anterior to the determination front, Mesp2-expressing cells occupy a domain that extends cephalically for the full length of the prospective new somite.[18] Mesp2 then induces expression of Ripply1 and Ripply2, which eliminate the Tbx6 protein over just that length. This displaces the expression of Tbx6 protein caudally into the presomitic mesoderm by exactly one somite length, so the new anterior border of Tbx6 defines the anterior border of the next somite to form.[29] Interactions between Mesp2 and Ripply2 then confer separate identities on the rostral and caudal halves of the newly forming somite, in preparation for the later cleavage of the somites and resegmentation into final segments.[30]

By these means, the boundary of the new somite forms at the anterior tip of the presomitic

mesoderm. There, the cells develop increased levels of adhesion molecules such as E-cadherin and neural cell adhesion molecule (NCAM). Mesp2 induces Eph-ephrin signaling activity, which participates in the epithelialization of somite boundary cells and defines the border between the newly forming somite and the anterior edge of the presomitic mesoderm behind it.[18] This process involves clustering of integrin alpha5 at the somite boundary, which in turn recruits fibronectin-based extracellular matrix to the forming border. The tissue mechanics involved in forming and defining the somite are reviewed in McMillen and Holley[31] (2015).[32]

Somite Symmetry

In vertebrates, RA helps to maintain symmetry between the developing somites.[1,3] Such symmetry is essential for later fusion of the left and right somites into symmetric vertebrae.[1]

Somite Differentiation

The newly formed epithelial somite immediately starts to mature and differentiate.[18] Cells in the ventral part of the somite deepithelialize to form the sclerotome, which then gives rise to (1) the vertebrae of the skeleton and (2) a thin layer of tendon progenitor cells designated the syndetome. This process is influenced by the levels of notochord-derived sonic hedgehog (Shh), which are highest in the ventral half-somite where Shh induces expression of paired box 1 (Pax1) and Pax9 in the sclerotome cells. In the dorsal portion of the somite, the dermomyotome cells remain epithelial. Wnt1/3a from the neural tube and Wnt8 from the ectoderm help induce expression of Pax3 and Pax7 in the dermomyotome. Cells from the tip of the dermomyotome then give rise to the underlying myotome, which starts to express myogenic factors Myf5 (myogenic factor 5) and MyoD (myogenic differentiation 1) and eventually generates the epiaxial (back) and hypaxial (body wall) muscles and part of the dermis of the back. Neurotrophin 3 (NTF3) from the neural tube induces specification of the dermatome, the precursor of dermis tissue.

Segment Number and Size

Species vary in the normal number of vertebral segments: frog, 10; human, 33; snake, more than 300.[33] In each, the mechanism of somitogenesis seems similar, with an anterior to posterior gradient of RA opposing a posterior to anterior gradient of FGF. In each, the regression speed of the MSGN1 anterior boundary during somitogenesis moves by 1 somite length during each period of somite formation, independent of the somitogenesis stage and the species.

AXIS TERMINATION

Toward the end of axial extension, the presomitic mesodermal domain decreases in size. Somitogenesis slows and then ceases, terminating axis extension. Amin and colleagues[34] propose that TBXT and Cdx2 stimulate axis extension by directly coactivating the Wnt and FGF growth signaling cascades in the progenitor niche and by activating the axial progenitors themselves. Then, activation of Hox13 genes downregulates TBXT and Cdx and thereby reduces Wnt and Fgf signaling in the growth zone. The Hox13 proteins also weaken the synergistic Cdx2/Hox trunk-stimulating loop at the trunk-to-tail transition in 2 ways. First, Hox13 proteins repress more anterior Hox genes, reducing the stimulation to growth, and second, they antagonize Cdx2 binding. These changes downregulate TBXT and Cdx, reduce Wnt and Fgf signaling in the growth zone, exhaust the neuromesodermal progenitors in their stem cell niche, and by depletion of progenitors, terminate elongation.[34] Other possible mechanisms involve BMP. In mice, FGF3 derived from the caudal presomitic mesoderm regulates BMP signal in the adjacent neuroepithelium. Increased BMP4 signaling depletes progenitors from the presomitic mesoderm, possibly providing an additional mechanism for slowing and termination of axis extension.[4]

JUNCTIONAL NEURULATION

Closure of the caudal neuropore and beginning of extension of the tailbud mark the end of primary neurulation and the onset of secondary neurulation. At the junction between the proximal portion of the spinal cord made by primary neurulation and the distal portion of the spinal cord made by secondary neurulation, the spinal cord is formed by a distinct developmental program designated junctional neurulation (Fig. 10).[35] This program requires coordinated movements of elevation and folding of the developing tube combined with ingression and accretion of cells to ensure topological continuity between the primary and secondary neural tube, while supplying all neural progenitors of both the junctional and secondary neural tube.[35]

During primary neurulation, the entire neural plate remains as an intact epithelium throughout the process of rolling, fold elevation, apposition, and fusion. The epithelial cells are all Sox2 positive, indicating that they are already committed to a neural fate. The basement membrane remains intact with no sign of breakdown. There are no signs of epithelial-mesenchymal transitions. However, in the junctional region, only the lateral cells show features of primary neural tube cells. The lateral cells are *Sox-2* positive (indicating commitment to neural fate), are organized as an epithelium, limited by a continuous basement membrane, and express E-cadherin. These cells ultimately contribute to the dorsal neural tube and undergo few major molecular changes, except a gradual E-cadherin to N-cadherin expression switch. In contrast, Sox-2–negative cells situated medially show features consistent with mesodermal progenitors. Initially, in the chick, at HH8, they are devoid of a basement membrane and show molecular markers of epithelial-mesenchymal transition. They then begin to express Sox-2 and mingle with the dorsolateral neural epithelial cells by a process resembling cell intercalation, followed by epithelialization and deposition of a basement membrane. Importantly, these initially Sox-2–negative cells contribute cells to the ventral neural tube in the junctional region and become a source of cells for the caudal neural tube generated by secondary neurulation. Thus, in the junctional region, the neural tube forms from 2 adjacent populations initially situated superficially,

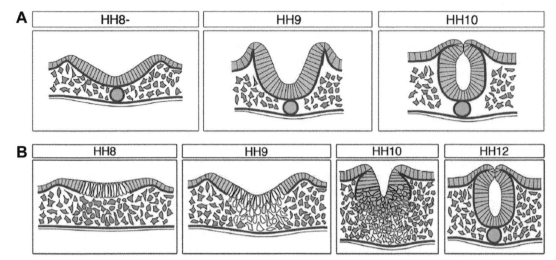

Fig. 10. Junctional neurulation. From left to right in each row, the panels indicate successive stages of neural tube formation from HH8 to HH12. (*Top*) Primary neurulation. Cross sections through the anterior trunk of the chick embryo at HH8–HH10. Formation of the primary neural tube is characterized by elevation of the neural folds and neural tube closure. In primary neurulation, the neural epithelium (*light blue*) remains as an intact epithelium with an intact basement membrane (*thick brown lines*) throughout the folding process until neural tube closure. Light blue, Sox-2–positive neural cells; light purple, ectoderm; green, notochord; orange, paraxial mesoderm. (*Bottom*) Cross sections through the node streak border at HH8–HH12, illustrating the movements of cell populations during formation of the junctional neural tube. At HH8, the superficial layer of the node streak border contains 2 adjacent cell populations: the lateral cell population contains Sox-2–positive neural cells that express E-cadherin and are limited by a basement membrane. The medial cell population contains Sox-2–negative cells with no basement membrane that are undergoing an E-cadherin to N-cadherin switch. From HH9 to HH12, the lateral cells undergo elevation and folding and are gradually displaced dorsally, as is seen during primary neurulation. The medial cells accumulate beneath the surface to form a mass of compact cells that progressively express Sox-2. These cells later reorganize as an epithelium in continuity with the dorsal neural tube and become limited by a basement membrane extending dorsoventrally. Light blue represents Sox-2–positive neural cells; white represents Sox-2–negative neural progenitors. (*From* Dady A et al. Junctional neurulation: a unique developmental program shaping a discrete region of the spinal cord highly susceptible to neural tube defects. The J of Neuroscience 2014;34(39):13208–13221. Fig. 4C page 13214 and 5C, page13215; with permission.)

but executing distinct morphogenetic programs before they assemble into a coherent neural tube. Because the overlap zone at the junction is oriented obliquely (**Fig. 11**), extending further caudally along the dorsal surface of the junction and further cephalically along the ventral surface, then, at the junction, cells arising from primary neural tube contribute more cells to the dorsal cord,

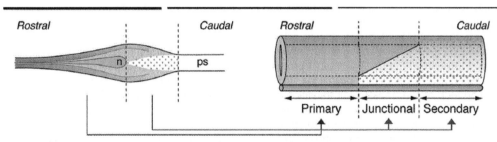

Fig. 11. Junctional neurulation. Topological continuity and overlap between the primary and secondary neural tubes in the node streak border. The node streak border at HH8 (*left*) and the resulting spinal cord (*right*) indicating the different populations that constitute the junctional zone at HH8 and their ultimate contribution to the neural tube along the rostrocaudal axis. Light blue, Sox-2–positive neural cells executing movements of primary neurulation; blue dots, Sox-2–negative neural progenitors undergoing epithelial-mesenchymal transition; green, notochord. n, Hensen node; ps, primitive streak. (*From* Dady A et al. Junctional neurulation: a unique developmental program shaping a discrete region of the spinal cord highly susceptible to neural tube defects. The J of Neuroscience 2014;34(39):13208–13221. Fig. 6F, page 13216; with permission.)

whereas cells arising from the secondary neural tube contribute more cells to the ventral cord.

SECONDARY NEURULATION

In humans, primary neurulation ends with the closure of the posterior neuropore opposite somites 30/31 at O'Rahilly and Müller stage 12. Distal to this, the caudal cell mass (tailbud) then gives rise to the caudal notochord, caudal somites, hind gut, and urogenital tracts in the caudal region of the embryo. Because human somites 30/31 correspond roughly to the S1-S2 junction, secondary neurulation gives rise to most of the sacrococcygeal spine, the conus, and the primordium for the filum terminale.

The specific process by which secondary neurulation proceeds has been debated, and compared, variably, with the chick or the mouse. In the mouse and other tailed animals, only the tail is made by secondary neurulation. In the chick, the anatomic region in which the spinal cord is shaped by secondary neurulation extends up to the lumbar region and matches more closely that found in humans. A junctional region in which primary neurulation overlaps dorsally with secondary neurulation is known in the chick and in humans, but not in the mouse.[35] It seems that the chick model more closely mimics the changes observed in humans.[36]

The human caudal cell mass first appears as a cluster of undifferentiated mesenchyme directly ventral to the receding primitive streak at stage 10.[36] This initially ill-defined mesenchymal mass enlarges rapidly and begins to serve as the source of cells for the caudal region during stage 12 when the caudal neural tube closes. Secondary neurulation proceeds through 3 distinct stages: (1) cellular aggregation and condensation to form a solid medullary cord; (2) cavitation of the medullary cord; and (3) partial regression and degeneration of the cavitary medullary cord to form the final structure. The following phases are seen in the chick:

1. Cellular aggregation and condensation phase: MET.[36] The early medullary cord emerges by cell sorting, in which the loose mesenchymal cells within the rostral portion of the secondary cord aggregate and elongate to form a compact rod of cells. The initially homogeneous rod then begins to display 2 different cell populations. A ring of peripheral cells begins to develop apicobasal orientation. Those cells develop intercellular tight junctions and become firmly adherent to each other. The apices of the cells point toward the center of the rod. Through intracellular nuclear shuffling, the peripheral cells develop into a pseudostratified epithelium. This transition (MET) from uncommitted mesenchyme to neural medullary cord epithelium is the most basic and important step in secondary neurulation.[36] Throughout this process, the central cells within the early medullary cord retain a loose, mesenchymal structure. With time, a distinct external limiting lamina forms on the basal (outer) side of the peripheral cells, surrounding the entire medullary cord. This lamina isolates the medullary cord from the surface ectoderm dorsally, from the caudal somites laterally, and from the prospective caudal notochord ventrally. The peripheral cells of the medullary cord ultimately contribute to the lateral walls of the secondary neural tube and show a morphology and radial arrangement identical to the neuroepithelium of the primary neural tube.[36]

2. Cavitation of the medullary cord.[36] As the cells within the early medullary cord begin to sort out, isolated small paracentral lumina form between the apices of the peripheral cells and the central cells. The central cells begin to disappear because of programmed apoptosis and/or intercalation into the peripheral epithelium. As the population of central cells decreases, the initially isolated paracentral lumina coalesce into a large central lumen. That lumen is lined by the apices of the radially oriented, peripheral, now-neuroepithelial cells, and the medullary cord takes on the appearance of the primary neural tube. The coalescence of the small lumina within the medullary cord occurs first at the junction between the primary and secondary cords. At that junction, there is a distinct overlap zone made up of the terminal portion of the primary neural tube dorsally and the most cranial (and youngest) portion of the medullary cord ventrally. The central canal of the primary neural tube merges with the now-single, coalescent canal of the secondary neural tube in the junctional, overlap zone to form a single seamless tube The 2 portions then continue to coalesce, craniocaudally, along the sequentially consolidating and cavitating medullary cord.

3. Degeneration of the medullary cord.[36] Once formed, the caudal portion of the secondary neural tissue begins to degenerate and undergo removal. In tailed animals, little needs to be removed. The tail gut must disappear, but most of the medullary cord, and all of the coccygeal vertebrae, remain as a functioning tail. In tailless mammals and avians, most of the medullary cord, coccygeal vertebrae, and somitic mesoderm regress. In humans the

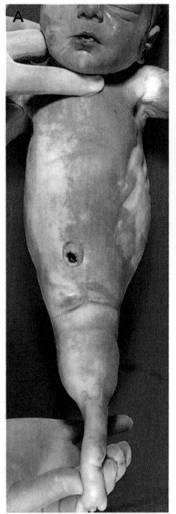

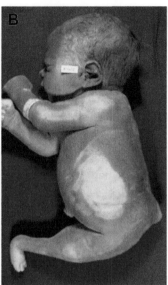

Fig. 12. Sirenomelia monopus. (*A*, *B*) Anterior and lateral views of a stillborn child with marked caudal hypoplasia, a single distal extremity, and a single foot. There is extreme hyperrotation of the lower extremity such that the knee bends anteriorly and the single foot points posteriorly. (*From* Naidich et al. Congenital anomalies of the spine and spinal cord. Chapter 24 pp. 1364-1447 [In] Scott W. Atlas Ed. Magnetic resonance imaging of the brain and spine. Fourth Ed. Vol 2. Philadelphia: Wolters Kluwer; 2009; with permission.)

medullary cord is reduced to the lower conus and the filum terminale. The tip of the caudal notochord degenerates with the exception of 1 or 2 pieces of coccygeal vertebrae. The tail gut distal to the cloacal membrane vanishes. In the chick, the base of the tail becomes incorporated into the caudal trunk.

ALTERED GENERATION OF MESODERM
Sirenomelia

The sirenomelia complex is a severe malformation of the caudal body characterized by apparent fusion of the legs into 1 lower "limb" (**Figs. 12** and **13**). The fusion of the lower extremities varies

from mild to severe. Concurrent lumbosacral and pelvic malformations include sacral agenesis, malformed vertebrae and hemivertebrae, with corresponding abnormalities of the central nervous system. Hindgut anomalies include blind-ending colon, rectal atresia, and imperforate anus. All human cases have variable degrees of renal and urethral dysplasia, commonly total renal agenesis. External genitalia are often absent or appear as an indistinct tag of tissue. Gonads are typically normal. The distal vasculature is abnormal. In the very few human babies who have survived, intelligence is normal.[10]

Sirenomelia is sporadic in humans but heritable in mice with defects in *brachyury* and in the *axin1*

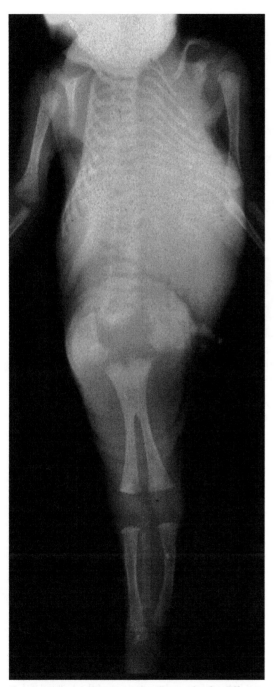

Fig. 13. Sirenomelia. Frontal radiograph of a different patient discloses paired partially fused femora, paired tibae, and a single thick midline fibula within the single lower extremity.

gene (related to β-catenin).[10] In mice, sirenomelia results from gain-of-function (excess) RA signaling, caused by defective Cyp26a1, the enzyme that breaks down RA in the caudal embryo. In addition, consistently, disruption of

Cdx2, which encodes a transcription factor that activates a promoter of *Cyp26a1* and disruption of *Por*, which encodes an enzyme required for Cyp26a1 function, also lead to sirenomelia in mice. Experimental administration of excess RA to pregnant mice leads to caudal malformations, including sirenomelia. Interestingly, Cyp26a1 normally participates in the formation of the distal vasculature, so disruption of Cyp26a1 signaling may also explain the abnormal vasculature in sirens. In mice, sirenomelia may also result from reduced BMP signaling in the caudal embryo. In zebrafish, deficient BMP signaling after the midgastrula stage causes deficient ventral mesoderm formation.[10]

ALTERED NEURULATION
Altered Primary Neurulation

Failure of primary neurulation leads to the series of open neural tube defects, most of which are characterized by incomplete closure of the tube in the dorsal midline (dorsal myeloschisis) and a wide variety of concurrent anomalies of the overlying soft tissue and bone. These open neural tube defects include the large group of overlapping craniovertebral anomalies designated anencephaly, cephalocele, and spinal dysraphism (see Jena L. Miller and Thierry A.G.M. Huisman's article, "Spinal Dysraphia, Chiari 2 Malformation, Unified Theory and Advances in Fetoscopic Repair," in this issue).

Altered Junctional Neurulation

Failure of junctional neurulation may lead to an ununited spinal cord composed of 2, physically separate, upper and lower segments made individually by primary and secondary neurulation (**Fig. 14**). Eibach and colleagues[37] (2017) and Schmidt and colleagues[38] (2017) reported a total of 4 such cases with clinical, imaging, and surgical features of failed junctional neurulation. There were 2 male and 2 female patients, newborn to 30 years of age, with no cutaneous stigmata. The 3 older patients presented at about 2 years of age with delayed ability to walk and complete urinary/fecal incontinence. In these 3 cases, the primary cord terminated between T11 and L1. The distal cord lay 3 to 5 spinal segments further caudally and, in each case, was connected to the primary cord only by a uniformly narrow band of tissue. This intervening band was functionally inert in the single case that underwent detailed neurophysiologic testing at surgery. In cases 1 to 3, the distal cord gave rise to multiple nerve roots bilaterally (sometimes a surplus of them) and tapered to a normal filum further caudally. Case 4 showed mild dilatation of the distal central canal

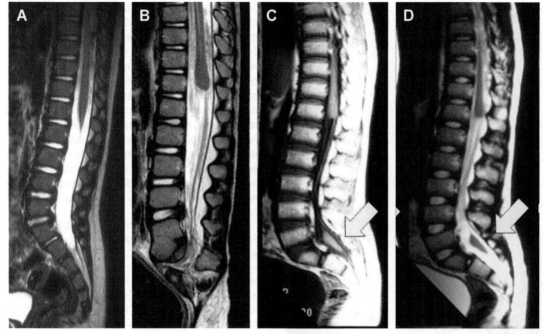

Fig. 14. The distal cord: normal versus malformation. (*A*) Normal. Midsagittal T2 magnetic resonance (MR) imaging shows the normal distal spinal column, conus medullaris, and thecal sac. (*B*) Caudal dysgenesis. Midsagittal T2 MR imaging shows chisel-shaped truncation of the distal cord that is similar to the portion of the primary neural tube that contributes to junctional neurulation (cf **Fig. 11**). There is partial sacral agenesis. (*C, D*) Failed junctional neurulation. Midsagittal T1 (*C*) and T2 (*D*) MR imaging show a truncated upper cord in abnormally high position (mid-T12) and a conical portion of neural tissue within the upper sacral canal (*arrows*).

of the proximal cord. Cases 1 and 3 had congenital scoliosis. Cases 1, 2, and 3 showed malsegmentation of thoracic and/or lumbar vertebrae, and 3 of the 4 cases showed distal sacral agenesis.

It is noted that the planar cell-polarity member, Prickle-1, is recruited specifically during junctional neurulation and its misexpression within a limited time period suffices to cause anomalies that phenocopy lower spine neural tube defects in humans.[35] Dady and colleagues[35] suggest that failed junctional neurulation phenocopies failed primary neurulation in the zone of overlap.

Altered Secondary Neurulation (Syndromes of Caudal Regression)

Truncation
Failure to form the secondary cord leaves a shortened, high-riding upper cord that may show a rounded termination or appear chisel shaped, with the dorsal sensory portion extending further caudally than the ventral motor portion (see **Fig. 14**B; **Fig. 15**).[30,39,40] There may be dilatation of the distal portion of the central canal of the cord. There are typically multiple concurrent

malformations of the spinal column, hind gut, and the distal urinary system.

Incomplete degeneration
Incomplete involution of the secondary cord leaves a long "neural" segment within the caudal spinal canal. Pang and colleagues[36] reported 7 cases of retained medullary cords, suggesting that such cords may have resulted from partial or complete arrest of secondary neurulation before or early in the degeneration phase. Such cases include the Currarino triad and partial sacral agenesis, which are well-recognized secondary neurulation defects. A terminal meningocele in their patient 5 also suggests a defect in the caudal paraxial mesoderm, which is derived from the caudal somites and is therefore a descendant of the tailbud.[36]

At surgery in these cases, the external appearance of the distal structure strongly resembled the spinal cord, with its expected diameter, color, pial covering, surface vasculature, and attendant nerve roots. Intraoperative stimulation of the distal cord and roots clearly delineated the end of the functional conus more superiorly, supporting the concept that the more distal, electrophysiologically silent portion is the part of the medullary cord that would have degenerated into a filum if

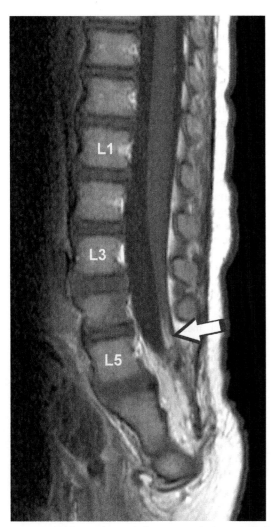

Fig. 15. Defect of secondary neurulation. Failed degeneration. Midsagittal T1 MR imaging shows incomplete involution of the secondary cord with gradual tapering of the low-lying primary cord into a spinal lipoma. The caudal spinal canal is dysplastic with distal sacral agenesis (*arrows*).

secondary neurulation had concluded properly. In one patient (number 4), a regular filum separated the normal conus from the distal medullary cord, suggesting that incomplete degeneration may affect just parts of the secondary cord.[36]

Internally, the medullary cord was found to be a pia-covered tube with a glial core containing disorganized clusters of neurons, surrounded by variable amounts of fat and fibrous tissue. In several specimens, parts of the core showed marginal-mantle layering as in a real spinal cord. The presence of 1, 2, or 3 nonconfluent ependymal-lined cavities within the medullary cord in 3 cases further suggests that the arrest of medullary involution occurred in the cavitation phase of

involution. This multicavitary pattern within the medullary cord evokes the pattern seen in the chick rather than the mouse model of secondary neurulation. The presence of mature glial cells and neurons in the surgical specimens suggests that the primitive secondary neuroepithelium in these medullary cords did undergo downstream differentiation, presumably because programmed dissolution had not taken place. None of the specimens showed evidence of apoptosis, but this could be a timing issue.[36]

Retained tail
At times, incomplete involution of the secondary cord leaves multiple dysplastic distal vertebral elements arrayed in an unusual shape, sometimes pointing dorsally. Pang and colleagues'[36] series included 1 such case.[36]

DEFECTS IN SOMITOGENESIS
Asymmetric Somitogenesis

Long after signaling sequences confer a definite left-right asymmetry for the internal organs such as heart and gut, somitogenesis establishes a series of now-symmetric vertebral and neural elements to form the normal spinal column and cord. In normal amniote embryos, RA helps to buffer the earlier-induced left-right bias and establish the bilaterally symmetric oscillations and segmentation that lead to normal symmetric somites.[26] In the absence of RA, the presomitic mesoderm is patterned by the asymmetrical signals that drive left-right differentiation of the body. Chicken, mouse, and fish embryos deprived of RA show asymmetrical somitogenesis, with somite formation consistently delayed on the left in chicks and on the right in zebrafish and mouse.[26] Experimentally, inverting the body situs inverts the side of delayed somitogenesis, indicating that the asymmetry is caused by the same machinery that controls asymmetric left-right development, downstream of Nodal signaling.[26] In zebrafish, repletion of RA leads to more rapid catch-up formation of somites in symmetric positions, whereas in mice the catch-up region may not be positioned symmetrically, or may even remain unpatterned.[26] These species-specific differences seem to result from alterations in the FGF8 gradient and from species-specific differences in somite boundary formation.[26]

Aberrant Somitogenesis

In humans, segmentation defects may arise from mutations in 4 similar genes that are known to be involved in the patterning of the presomitic mesoderm (LFNG, MESP2, HES7, and deltalike 3

[DLL3]).[18] In mice, mutations in the Notch signaling pathway may lead to spondylocostal dysostosis.[13] Disorders of the RA gradient, endogenous or exogenous, shift the identities of individual vertebrae, altering the relative numbers of cervical, thoracic, lumbar, and sacral vertebrae. Variation in RA in utero may explain the transitional vertebrae seen in 2% to 6% of the population.

In mouse, eliminating or reducing Notch signaling results in disrupted somite boundaries and disordered hes/her gene expression, but not complete absence of somites or loss of all hes/her gene expression. It seems that Notch signaling only modulates the timing of *hes/her* gene oscillation and thereby leads to synchronization of neighboring presomitic mesodermal cells.[19] In fish, the rate of somitogenesis can vary 3-fold over a 10° temperature range. However, the total number of somites and somite length show minor to no change over this temperature range. These findings suggest that somitogenesis precisely compensates for the variations in elongation rate caused by temperature fluctuation.[17]

PHYLOGENY

Evolutionarily, Cdx and Hox genes both derive from an ancient protoHox gene or gene cluster.[12] With wear and tear, the 4 human Hox clusters are variably complete, containing some 9 to 11 of the original 13 genes in each cluster. Hox A is the most nearly complete, missing only Hox A8 and A12[34] Genes missing from the other three clusters are B10, B11 and B12; C1, C2, C3 and C7; and D2, D5, D6 and D7.[34]

There are substantial evolutionary differences in somitogenesis among species.[26] In some species, RA is not necessary for somite formation. In amphioxus, somitogenesis is asymmetric, and FGF8 is not required for the formation of the posterior somites. FGF and RA do not interact, and RA is not able to generate symmetric somitogenesis. It thus seems that the FGF-RA antagonism may have evolved to ensure symmetric somitogenesis in vertebrates.[26]

Brachyury has also been shown to help establish the cervical vertebral blueprint during fetal development. The number of cervical vertebrae is highly conserved among all mammals. All but 3 known mammalian genera have a strictly conserved pattern of 7 cervical vertebrae. A spontaneous mutation in the Brachyury gene in the cow (*Bos taurus*) has been found to cause vertebral and spinal dysplasia, which includes a reduced number of cervical vertebrae. Thus, Brachyury is directly involved in the maintenance of the mammalian 7 cervical vertebrae.[41]

SUMMARY

The intricate mechanisms by which the distal spine and spinal cord are generated and the many variations in the malformations related to them are a fascinating and lifelong study. After decades of study of phenotypes, such as sirenomelia, elucidation of the mechanism of malformation is deeply satisfying, and inspires hope that, one day, increased understanding and improved technology may enable clinicians to improve diet to avoid such malformations and to detect and treat them in utero when they do occur.

REFERENCES

1. Aulehla A, Pourquié O. Signaling gradients during paraxial mesoderm development. Cold Spring Harb Perspect Biol 2010;2:a000869.
2. Balasubramanian R, Zhang X. Mechanisms of FGF gradient formation during embryogenesis. Semin Cell Dev Biol 2016;53:94–100.
3. Diez del Corral R, Morale AV. The multiple roles of FGF signaling in the developing spinal cord. Front Cell Dev Biol 2017. https://doi.org/10.3389/fcell. 2017.00058.
4. Anderson MJ, Schimmang T, Lewandoski M. An FGF3-BMP signaling axis regulates caudal neural tube closure, neural crest specification and anterior-posterior axis extension. PLoS Genet 2016; 12(5):e1006018.
5. Bejsovec A. Wingless signaling: a genetic journey from morphogenesis to metastasis. Genetics 2018; 208:1311–36.
6. MacDonald BT, Tamai K, He X. Wnt/B-catenin signaling: component, mechanisms and diseases. Dev Cell 2009;17(1):9–26.
7. Gao C, Xiao G, Hu J. Regulation of Wnt/β-catenin signaling by post translational modifications. Cell Biosci 2014;4:13.
8. Deschamps J, Duboule D. Embryonic timing, axial stem cells, chromatin dynamics and the Hox clock. Genes Dev 2017;31:1406–16.
9. Metzis V, Steinhauser S, Pakanavicius E, et al. Nervous system regionalization entails axial allocation before neural differentiation. Cell 2018; 175:1105–18.
10. Garrido-Allepuz C, Haro E, González-Lamuño D, et al. A clinical and experimental overview of sirenomelia: insight into the mechanisms of congenital limb malformations. Dis Model Mech 2011;4(3):289–99.
11. Katagiri T, Watabe T. Bone morphogenetic proteins. Cold Spring Harb Perspect Biol 2016;8:a021899.

12. Neijts R, Deschamps J. At the base of colinear Hox gene expression: cis-features and trans-factors orchestrating the initial phase of Hox cluster activation. Dev Biol 2017;428:293–9.

13. Wahi K, Bochter MS, Cole SE. The many roles of Notch signaling during vertebrate somitogenesis. Semin Cell Dev Biol 2016;49:68–75.

14. Dixon JR, Selvaraj S, Yue F, et al. Topological domains in mammalian genomes identified by analysis of chromatin interactions. Nature 2012;485(7398):376–80.

15. Zhu K, Spaink HP, Durston AJ. Collinear Hox-Hox interactions are involved in patterning the vertebrate anteroposterior (A-P) axis. PLoS One 2017. https://doi.org/10.1371/journal.pone.0175287.

16. Neijts R, Amin S, van Rooijen C, et al. Cdx is crucial for the timing mechanism driving collinear Hox activation and defines a trunk segment in the Hox cluster topology. Dev Biol 2017;422:146–54.

17. Liao B-K, Oates AC. Delta-Notch signaling in segmentation. Arthropod Struct Dev 2017;46:429–47.

18. Maroto M, Bone RA, Dale JK. Somitogenesis. Development 2012;139:2453–6.

19. Oates AC, Morelli LG, Ares S. Patterning embryos with oscillations: structure, function and dynamics of the vertebrate segmentation clock. Development 2012;139:625–39.

20. Bénazéraf B. Dynamics and mechanisms of posterior axis elongation of the vertebrate embryo. Cell Mol Life Sci 2019;76:89–98.

21. Chalamalasetty RB, Garriock RJ, Dunty WC Jr, et al. Mesogenin 1 is a master regulator of paraxial presomitic mesoderm differentiation. Development 2014;141:4285–97.

22. Gouti M, Metzis V, Briscoe J. The route to spinal cord cell types: a tale of signals and switches. Trends Genet 2015;31(6):282–9.

23. Gouti M, Tsakiridis A, Wymeersch FJ, et al. *In Vitro* generation of neuromesodermal progenitors reveals distinct roles for Wnt signaling in the specification of spinal cord and paraxial mesoderm identity. PLoS Biol 2014;12(8):e1001937.

24. Hubaud A, Pourquié O. Signalling dynamics in vertebrate segmentation. Nat Rev Mol Cell Biol 2014;15:709–21.

25. Martin BL. Factors that coordinate mesoderm specification from neuromesodermal progenitors with segmentation during vertebrate axis extension. Semin Cell Dev Biol 2016;49:59–67.

26. Vroomans RMA, ten Tusscher KHWJ. Modelling asymmetric somitogenesis: Deciphering the mechanisms behind species differences. Dev Biol 2017;427:21–34.

27. Niwa Y, Shimojo H, Isomura A, et al. Different types of oscillations in Notch and Fgf signaling regulate the spatiotemporal periodicity of somitogenesis. Genes Dev 2011;25(11):1115–20.

28. Sonnen KF, Lauschke VM, Uraji J, et al. Modulation of phase shift between Wnt and notch signaling oscillations controls mesoderm segmentation. Cell 2018;172:10079–1090.

29. Morimoto M, Sasaki N, Oginuma M, et al. The negative regulation of Mesp2 by mouse Ripply2 is required to establish the rostro-caudal patterning within a somite. Development 2007;134(8):1561–9.

30. Yabe T, Takada S. Molecular mechanism for cyclic generation of somites: Lessons from mice and zebrafish. Dev Growth Differ 2016;58(1):31–42.

31. McMillen P, Holley SA. The tissue mechanics of vertebrate body elongation and segmentation. Curr Opin Genet Dev 2015;32:106–11.

32. Merello E, De Marco P, Mascelli S, et al. HLXB9 homeobox gene and caudal regression syndrome. Birth Defects Res A Clin Mol Teratol 2006;76:205–9.

33. Gomez C, Özbudak EM, Wunderlich J, et al. Control of segment number in vertebrate embryos. Nature 2008;454:335–9.

34. Amin S, Neijts R, Simmini S, et al. Cdx and T brachyury co-activate growth signaling in the embryonic axial progenitor niche. Cell Rep 2016;17:3165–77.

35. Dady A, Havis E, Escriou V, et al. Junctional neurulation: a unique developmental program shaping a discrete region of the spinal cord highly susceptible to neural tube defects. J Neurosci 2014;34(39):13208–21.

36. Pang D, Zovickian J, Moes GS. Retained medullary cord in humans: late arrest of secondary neurulation. Neurosurgery 2011;68(6):1500–19.

37. Eibach S, Moes G, Hou YJ, et al. Unjoined primary and secondary neural tubes: junctional neural tube defect, a new form of spinal dysraphism caused by a disturbance of junctional neurulation. Childs Nerv Syst 2017;33:1633–47.

38. Schmidt C, Voin V, Iwanaga J, et al. Junctional neural tube defect in a newborn: report of a fourth case. Childs Nerv Syst 2017;33:873–5.

39. Cunningham TJ, Colas A, Duester G. Early molecular events during retinoic acid induced differentiation of neuromesodermal progenitors. Biol Open 2016;5:1821–33.

40. Currarino G, Coln R, Votteler T. Triad of anorectal, sacral, and presacral anomalies. AJR Am J Roentgenol 1981;137:395–8.

41. Kromik A, Ulrich R, Kusenda M, et al. The mammalian cervical vertebrae blueprint depends on the T (*brachyury*) Gene. Genetics 2015;199:873–83.

Disorders of Ventral Induction/Spectrum of Holoprosencephaly

Sonia Francesca Calloni, MD[a],*, Luca Caschera, MD[b],
Fabio Maria Triulzi, MD[c]

KEYWORDS

- Holoprosencephaly • Syntelencephaly • Magnetic resonance • Brain • Neurodevelopment
- Ventral induction

KEY POINTS

- The commonly seen disorders of ventral induction include holoprosencephaly, atelencephaly, agenesis of the corpus callosum, and agenesis of the septum pellucidum (septo-optic dysplasia).
- Holoprosencephaly results from the incomplete midline cleavage of the prosencephalon. It is classically divided into four types: alobar, semilobar, lobar form, and the middle interhemispheric variant, the latter also known as syntelencephaly.
- Septo-optic dysplasia features absence of the septum pellucidum in association with optic nerve abnormalities and/or pituitary dysfunction.

INTRODUCTION

Disorders of ventral induction include a group of conditions characterized by the anomalous process of cleavage of the brain and formation of midline structures, resulting in a wide spectrum of severity. The process of ventral induction takes place between the fifth week after conception and midgestation: insults during this phase affect the development of brain vesicles and the formation of the facial skeleton, their severity being closely related with the time of occurrence. Based on the embryologic brain development, these pathologic conditions are divided in disorders of prosencephalic cleavage, such as holoprosencephaly (HPE) and atelencephaly, and disorders of prosencephalic midline development, resulting in agenesis of the corpus callosum, agenesis of septum pellucidum, and septo-optic dysplasia (SOD).

Abnormalities of the prosencephalic formation are represented by aprosencephaly and atelencephaly, but are extremely rare. This article focuses on the different forms of HPE and SOD. Agenesis of the corpus callosum is extensively discussed elsewhere in this issue.

EMBRYOLOGY

The anterior neuropore, located at the most rostral end of the neural tube, closes approximately on embryonic day 25. Subsequently dramatic changes in morphology lead to the formation of the three primary brain vesicles, which from anterior to posterior include the prosencephalon, the mesencephalon, and the rhomboencephalon. By the end of the embryonic period, which in humans extends through gestational week 8 that corresponds approximately to embryonic day 49, these

Disclosure Statement: The authors have nothing to disclose.
[a] Department of Neuroradiology, San Raffaele Scientific Institute, Via Olgettina Milano 60, 20132 Milano, Italy; [b] Post-graduation School in Radiodiagnostic, University of Milan, Via Festa Del Perdono 9, 20122 Milano, Italy; [c] Neuroradiology Unit, Fondazione IRCCS Ca' Granda Ospedale Maggiore Policlinico, Via Francesco Sforza 35, 20122 Milano, Italy
* Corresponding author.
E-mail address: calloni.soniafrancesca@hsr.it

neuroimaging.theclinics.com

three segments further subdivide into five secondary brain vesicles. The prosencephalon divides into telencephalon and diencephalon, the rhomboencephalon divides into the metencephalon and myelencephalon. A subsequent partitioning of the telencephalic vesicle into two hemispheres follows, leading to the formation of the interhemispheric fissure (Carnegie stage 16, embryonic day 32) and the differentiation of the falx cerebri (Carnegie stages 22–23, embryonic day 56),caused by the induction by bone morphogenetic proteins along the midline roof plate.[1] Their differentiation occurs before the neural tube closes.

HOLOPROSENCEPHALY

HPE (Mendelian Inheritance in Man [MIM] 236100) is a complex brain malformation resulting from incomplete cleavage of the prosencephalon into the right and left hemispheres, occurring between the 18th and the 28th day of gestation. HPE has a worldwide distribution, and its prevalence is estimated to be 1/10,000 live. There is a reported female preponderance 3:1 in alobar and 1:1 in lobar HPE.[2]

Etiology and Genetics

The causes of HPE include environmental factors, such as maternal diabetes mellitus (1% risk corresponding to a 200-fold increase compared with the general population)[3]; alcohol and retinoic acid use (although without established significance in humans)[4]; maternal hypocholesterolemia[5]; and genetic factors (approximately 25%–50% of cases, 13 trisomy the most common). Among heritable causes, cytogenetic abnormalities (numeric chromosome abnormalities and structural chromosome abnormalities), molecular abnormalities (copy number variants), and single gene pathogenic variants (syndromic HPE and nonsyndromic HPE) are recognized. Cytogenetic abnormalities causing HPE are more likely to manifest with other organ system involvement,[6] whereas nonsyndromic forms of HPE are the best understood at a molecular level and are inherited in an autosomal-dominant manner.[7] At least 14 mutated genes have been associated with autosomal-dominant nonsyndromic HPE, the most common being Sonic Hedgeog (SHH; 30%–40%) located on chromosome 7q36 and ZIC2 (5%) located on chromosome 13q32. Three involved genes belong to the Sonic Hedgehog pathway (SHH, PTCH-1, GLI2). Sonic hedgehog is a diffusible protein involved in establishing cell fates at several points during development. After being translocated from the cellular cytoplasm

into the extracellular space it binds to and acts as inhibitor of the membrane receptor Patched-1; such inhibition results in the relieve of the target membrane receptor Smoothened (SMO) otherwise antagonized by Patched-1. Smoothened activation is intracellularly mediated by the cytoplasmic proteins Gli1, Gli2, and Gli3 that subsequently translocate into the nucleus where they act as transcriptor factors. SHH is normally expressed, among other tissues, in the prechordal mesoderm and its mutation or the mutation of genes encoding for proteins down its pathway gives rise to a disorder of ventral induction and partitioning of the telencephalic vescicles.[7] However, ZIC2 gene is expressed in the dorsal neural tube suggesting that these two proteins may affect neural development in different ways. It encodes for a zinc finger gene homologous to the odd-paired gene of Drosophila and its mutations leads to HPE without any craniofacial involvement.[8] Other genes are rarely reported to be associated with autosomal-dominant nonsyndromic HPE: SIX3 (2p21), TGIF1 (18p11.3), GLI2 (2q14), PTCH1 (9q22.3), DISP1 (1q42), FGF8 (10q24), FOXH1 (8q24.3), NODAL (10q22.1), TDGF1 (3p23-p21), GAS1 (9q21.33), DLL1 (6q27), and CDON (11q24.2). Syndromic forms of HPE (18%–25%) have been occasionally reported in at least 25 different conditions categorized by mode of inheritance[9]: autosomal-dominant (Pallister-Hall syndrome, Rubinstein-Taybi syndrome, Kallmann syndrome with isolated gonadotropin-releasing hormone deficiency, Martin syndrome, Steinfeld syndrome, Hartsfield syndrome),[10] autosomal-recessive (Smith-Lemli-Opitz syndrome,[11] Meckel syndrome, Genoa syndrome, Lambotte syndrome, hydrolethalus syndrome, facial clefts, and brachial amelia), and unknown mode of inheritance (caudal dysgenesis).[12]

Clinical and Imaging Findings

Classic HPE encompasses a continuum of brain malformations classified by DeMyer and Zeman[13] following anatomic characteristics and clinical severity: alobar, semilobar, and lobar type. This classification is primarily based on the presence or absence of the interhemispheric fissure separating the two cerebral hemispheres and the extent of the fissure. Another milder subtype of HPE called the middle interhemispheric variant (MIH), or syntelencephaly, has now been recognized. Barkovich and colleagues[14] observed diffuse and focal abnormal sulci in most cases, subcortical heterotopia being the only malformation of cortical development to be usually found. They suggested that assessing and measuring the sylvian fissure angle may help in quantifying the severity of HPE: the greater the sylvian angle is, the more severe the HPE.

Diagnosis is made by prenatal ultrasound (US) between 10 and 14 weeks based on abnormal facial morphology and absence of the so called "butterfly sign," created by the two choroid plexus that are normally narrow in the middle but thicker at both ends and that resembles a butterfly's wings.[15] By the time of the second-trimester scan, the diagnosis of alobar HPE should be unequivocal. Radiologists and sonographers should always pay attention to the cavum septum pellucidum, which represents a hallmark in all severities of HPE: the accurate assessment of its presence and correct development is vital to detect milder forms, especially if facial abnormality is absent.[16]

If a normal cavum septum pellucidum is not detectable on routine US images, careful follow-up is essential with three-dimensional volume acquisition by vaginal US, which helps assessing the ventricular system directly. MR imaging allows to better define neuroanatomy in case of confusing or questionable US findings. Abnormal white matter maturation/myelination can also be depicted in better detail by MR imaging.[14]

HPE is accompanied by a spectrum of characteristic craniofacial anomalies, ranging from mild (choanal stenosis, pyriform sinus stenosis, hypotelorism, solitary maxillary median incisor) to severe forms (cyclopia, proboscis, cleft lip/palate, coloboma, retinal dysplasia). Severe forms (especially in the presence of a chromosomal anomaly) are often fatal and mortality is correlated with the severity of brain malformation and associated defects. Clinical manifestations in surviving children include motor and developmental delay, hydrocephalus, epilepsy, and oromotor and hypothalamic dysfunction.[9] Table 1 summarizes major facial dysmorphism and imaging findings.

Alobar Holoprosencephaly

In alobar HPE there is a complete prosencephalic cleavage failure, thus resulting in a single midline forebrain with a primitive ventricle. A large dorsal cyst is typically present in alobar HPE, much less frequently in semilobar HPE and lobar HPE (92%, 28%, and 9%, respectively).[17] Among the types, alobar HPE is the most frequent type, ranging between 40% and 75%.[2] The affected fetus often dies intrauterine or soon after birth, or during the first 6 months of life. US in the antenatal period reveals a monoventricle, fused thalami and basal ganglia, absence of the corpus callosum and anterior commissure, and absence of the cavum septum pellucidum, and of course no interhemispheric fissure.[16] According to Paladini and Volpe[18] fused cerebral cortex can resemble three different shapes on sagittal views: (1) pancake-like, (2) cup-like, and (3) ball-like. In the pancake-like, cerebral tissue is confined to the basicranium, squeezed by the large cyst. In the cup-like shape cerebral tissue covers variable amounts of the anterior cranium with a dorsal cyst present posteriorly. In the ball-like, a complete rim of tissue surrounds the monoventricle without dorsal cyst. In alobar HPE cerebral and middle and the anterior artery do not develop in almost all cases, and are replaced by tangled vessels arising from the internal carotid and basilar vessels.[19] On midsagittal view anterior cerebral artery lies underneath the frontal bone resembling a "snake under the skull," which is another typical US sign for this brain disorder. The gyral pattern is disorganized.[20] The optic nerves may be absent, present, or fused.[21] Fetal MR imaging does not add much to the US findings in alobar HPE, because it is mostly useful to discriminate subtle forms of the spectrum (Fig. 1).[22] A cytoarchitectonic analysis recently indicated that the area of frontal cortex normally located just anteriorly to the motor strip is never induced to form in alobar HPE. This is consistent with the current theory of the embryogenesis of HPE, which postulates a defect in dorsoventral patterning at the most rostral end of the neural tube.[20]

Semilobar Holoprosencephaly

The correct identification of a semilobar HPE from the other forms is challenging, and the absence of the septum pellucidum is typically the only hint at the 18- to 20-week US examination.[23] Facial malformations are usually absent or mild, the most common being hypotelorism and cleft lip.[24] Classic imaging findings are rudimentary lobes and a monoventricle with partially developed occipital and temporal horns. The interhemispheric fissure is only present posteriorly. The correct development of the anterior portion of the corpus callosum depends on a well-developed interhemispheric fissure. The substrate underlying the early callosal tract crossing the midline through the interhemispheric fissure are known to be comprised of astroglial cells that express the marker Gfap, the so-called midline zipper glia.[25] Recent studies demonstrated that the midline zipper glia remodels the interhemispheric fissure before callosal tract formation.[26,27] The anterior portion of the corpus callosum (genu and anterior

Table 1
Radiologic findings and correlated facial dysmorphisms for the four types of HPE

Type of HPE	Imaging Findings	Facial Dysmorphism
Alobar	Small monoventricle No interhemispheric division Absence of olfactory bulbs and tracts Absence of corpus callosum Fusion of deep gray nuclei	Cyclopia without proboscis Ethmocephaly Cebocephaly Closely spaced eyes Anophthalmia or microphthalmia Premaxillary agenesis with median cleft lip, closely spaced eyes, depressed nasal ridge Bilateral cleft lip Relatively normal facial appearance (especially in persons with pathogenic variants in *ZIC2*)
Semilobar	Rudimentary cerebral lobes Partially developed occipital and temporal horns Incomplete interhemispheric division (only posteriorly) Absence or hypoplasia of olfactory bulbs and tracts Absence of corpus callosum Varying nonseparation of deep gray nuclei (fusion of the thalami)	Closely spaced eyes Anophthalmia/microphthalmia Depressed nasal bridge Absent nasal septum Flat nasal tip Bilateral cleft lip with median process representing the philtrum-premaxilla anlage Midline cleft (lip and/or palate) Relatively normal facial appearance
Lobar	Fully developed cerebral lobes Distinct interhemispheric division Midline continuous frontal neocortex Callosal genu and splenium hypoplastic Fused fornix Septum pellucidum possibly absent	Bilateral cleft lip with median process Closely spaced eyes Depressed nasal ridge Relatively normal facial appearance
MIH	Failure of separation of the posterior frontal and parietal lobes Callosal genu and splenium normally formed Absence of corpus callosum Hypothalamus and lentiform nuclei normally separated Caudate nuclei and thalami partially fused Heterotopic gray matter Cerebellar anomalies	Closely spaced eyes Depressed nasal bridge Narrow nasal bridge Relatively normal facial appearance

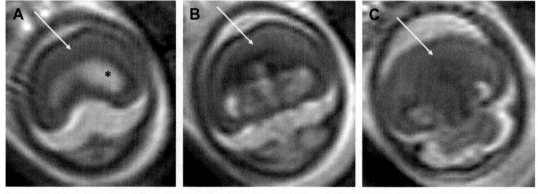

Fig. 1. (*A–C*) Fetal MR imaging at 21 gestational weeks; single shot fast spin echo (SSFSE) T2-weighted images at three different axial cuts from the vertex downward demonstrate complete failure of separation of the two cerebral hemispheres (*arrow*) resulting in a single midline forebrain with a primitive monoventricle (*asterisk*).

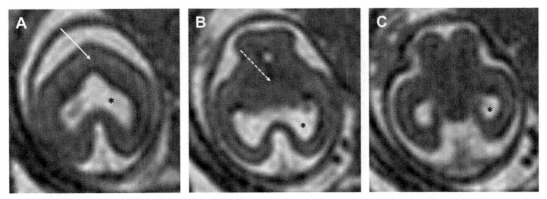

Fig. 2. (A–C) Fetal MR imaging at 21 gestational weeks; fast field echo T2-weighted images at three different axial cuts from the vertex downward demonstrate almost complete failure of separation of the two cerebral hemispheres (*solid arrow*), absence of the septum pellucidum, rudimentary lobes with fusion of the thalami (*dotted arrow*), and a monoventricle with partially developed occipital and temporal horns (*asterisk*).

body) is always absent; the splenium is typically normally developed in semilobar HPE.[28] Olfactory bulbs and tracts are also absent or hypoplastic. Deep gray nuclei can also be partially fused, especially the thalami. Gyral pattern is usually disorganized (**Fig. 2**).

Lobar Holoprosencephaly

Lobar HPE is the mildest of the three forms. It is characterized by an almost complete separation of the cerebral hemispheres and deep gray matter nuclei except for the most rostral frontal lobes. The genu of the corpus callosum is mildly hypoplastic or dysplastic. A fused fornix is demonstrated by US as an echogenic linear structure running anteroposterior within the third ventricle, but this findings can also be consistent with other midline brain abnormalities including SOD.[29] The olfactory bulbs and sulci are usually normal or mildly hypoplastic. The ventricular system is unremarkable in morphology, although the septum pellucidum is often absent (**Fig. 3**).[28] Despite the presence of an apparent interhemispheric fissure, cerebral cortex is still found crossing the midline along virtually the entire anterior-posterior axis.[20]

Middle-Interhemispheric Variants

The MIH variant, also known as syntelencephaly, is a mild subtype of HPE, firstly described by Barkovich and Quint.[30] About 2% to 15% of HPE patients have MIH type. ZIC2 gene, on chromosome

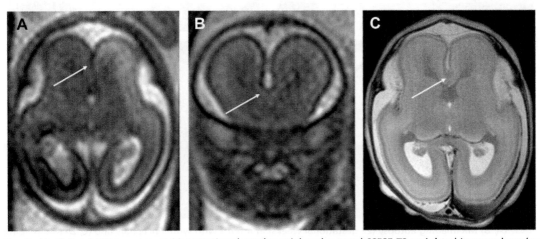

Fig. 3. (A, B) Fetal MR imaging at 20 gestational weeks; axial and coronal SSFSE T2-weighted images show (*arrow*) anterior fusion of the frontal lobes with continuity of the cortical plate along the midline. (C) MR imaging autopsy at 21 gestational weeks of the same case showed in A and B; axial turbo spin echo (TSE) T2-weighted image shows more clearly (*arrow*) the lack of anterior midline separation of the frontal lobes.

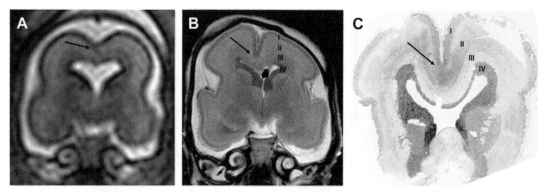

Fig. 4. (A) Fetal MR imaging at 20 + 5 gestational weeks; coronal SSFSE weighted image shows midline continuity (*arrow*) of the cerebral hemispheres at the level of posterior frontal and parietal regions. (B) MR imaging autopsy at 22 gestational weeks of the same case showed in A; coronal TSE T2-weighted image shows more clearly (*arrow*) the lack of separation between the two hemispheres with continuity of the cortical plate along the midline. (C) Paraffin-embedded formalin-fixed hematoxylin and eosin stained coronal cut of the same patients depicted in A and B; cortical plate (*arrow*) is continuous along the midline determining an abnormal midline connection of the cerebral hemispheres. I, cortical plate; II, subplate; III, intermediate zone; IV, germinal zone.

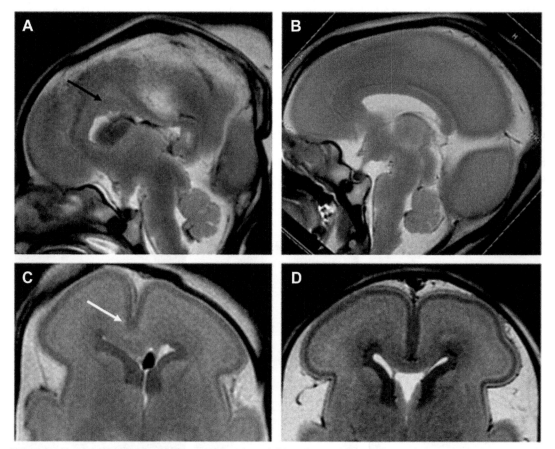

Fig. 5. (A, B) MR imaging autopsy (22 gestational weeks) in a fetus with syntelencephaly and (C, D) MR imaging autopsy of a normal brain fetus for comparison. (A) Sagittal TSE T2-weighted image shows (*black arrow*) an abnormal midline connection of the cerebral hemispheres in the posterior frontal and parietal regions, with interhemispheric separation of the basal forebrain, anterior frontal lobes, and occipital regions. (C) Coronal TSE T2-weighted image shows (*white arrow*) continuity of the cortical plate along the midline.

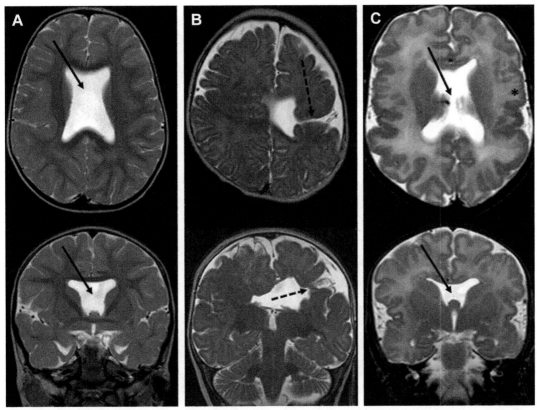

Fig. 6. Axial and coronal SSFSE T2-weighted images of three different patients with abnormalities included in the spectrum of septo-optic-dysplasia. (*A*) MR imaging of a 20-month-old patient demonstrates apparent isolated absence of the septum pellucidum (*arrow*). (*B*) MR imaging of a 7-month-old patient demonstrates absence of the septum pellucidum associated with open lip schizencephaly (*dotted arrow*) configuring a case of SOD plus. (*C*) MR imaging at 16 days after birth demonstrates absence of septum pellucidum (*arrow*) associated with diffuse abnormal gyration (*asterisk*) and white matter hyperintensity.

13q32, is known to be important in regulating neural tube closure and in promoting the embryonic roof plate differentiation. Mutations in this gene have been recognized as a potential cause of MIH. In MIH the posterior frontal and parietal lobes fail to split, often with the sylvian fissure passing coronally over the vertex of the connected brain to join with the fissure from the other side, documented by US.[31] The anteroinferior portion of the prosencephalon has a normal development, resulting in regular formation of the inferior frontal lobes, lentiform nuclei, and hypothalamic nuclei, whereas the caudate nuclei and thalami are often incompletely separated. Dorsal cyst is seen, but much less frequently than in other forms (Figs. 4 and 5). Cerebellar abnormalities and polymicrogyria are usually associated. MR imaging usually reveal a normal or mildly dysplastic anterior falx, whereas the posterior aspect is absent. The most typical finding is the absence of the body of the corpus callosum, whereas the splenium and

the genu are present. An azygous anterior cerebral artery is also noted in most cases.[32] Clinical findings are related to involvement of the motor cortex, including spasticity or hypotonia, and oromotor deficits.[32]

SEPTO-OPTIC DYSPLASIA

The typical SOD (MIM 182230) was first described histologically in 1956 by De Morsier.[33] It is a variable disorder characterized by any combination of the following findings: (1) optic nerve hypoplasia; (2) pituitary hypofunction; and (3) midline brain abnormalities, typically dysgenesis of the septum pellucidum and/or corpus callosum, or hypoplasia of the pons, of the vermis, and of the medulla.[34] There is a reported incidence of 1 in 10,000 live births.[35] Approximately 30% of all SOD patients have the full manifestation.[36] The septum pellucidum is interposed between the corpus callosum and the body of the fornix and should be

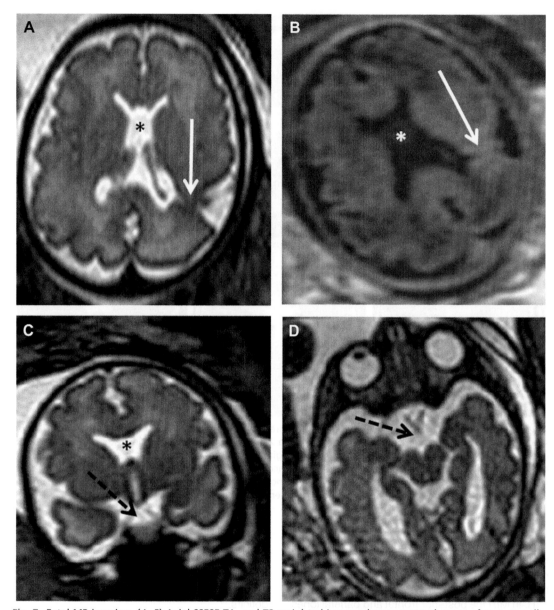

Fig. 7. Fetal MR imaging. (*A, B*) Axial SSFSE T1- and T2-weighted images demonstrate absence of septum pellucidum (*asterisk*) and closed lip schizencephaly (*solid arrow*). (*C, D*) Coronal and axial SSFSE-weighted images demonstrate absent of septum pellucidum (*asterisk*) and hypoplasia of the optic chiasm (*dotted arrow*).

considered connected with them. To date, several early developmental transcription factors and genes have been implicated in the cause of SOD: HESX1, SOX2, SOX3, OTX2, PROKR2, FGF1, and FGF8.[37] Mutations in these genes result in a heterogenous pattern of clinical and phenotypic presentations, because they are connected to the development of the forebrain and related midbrain structures.[34] Other risk factors have been implicated in its pathogenesis, such as maternal diabetes, antiepileptics, drug and alcohol abuse, and cytomegalovirus infection.[35]

Individuals with SOD can have different grades of pituitary-hypothalamic dysfunction, and variable neurodevelopmental outcomes, from normal cognition and development to developmental delay, autism, and epilepsy.[38] The main distinction in the clinical scenario is made by the presence or absence of schizencephaly, meaning a gray matter lined cleft extending from the ependyma to the pia mater. Precocious puberty, short stature, sleep problems, obesity, lack of smell (anosmia), hearing loss, and heart anomalies can also be present. When assessing

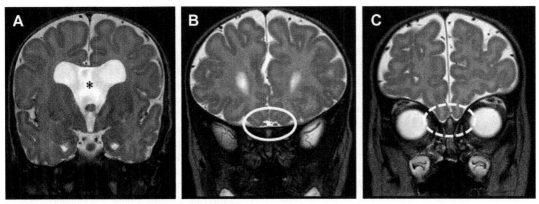

Fig. 8. (*A–C*) Coronal SSFSE T2-weighted images at three different coronal cuts obtained progressively from back to front of a 3-month-old patient demonstrates absence of septum pellucidum (*asterisk*), presence of the olfactory nerves (*circle*), but aplasia of the olfactory bulbs at the level of the olfactory fossae (*dotted circle*).

SOD, MR imaging is the imaging of choice: it shows the absence of the septum pellucidum, which results in a boxlike shape of the lateral ventricles on coronal imaging, the bilateral frontal horns appearing squared off. Abnormalities of the optic nerves and chiasm are well depicted by MR imaging. Pituitary gland malformations include anterior pituitary hypoplasia, ectopic posterior lobe, and/or thin or interrupted pituitary stalk (**Figs. 6–9**).[39,40]

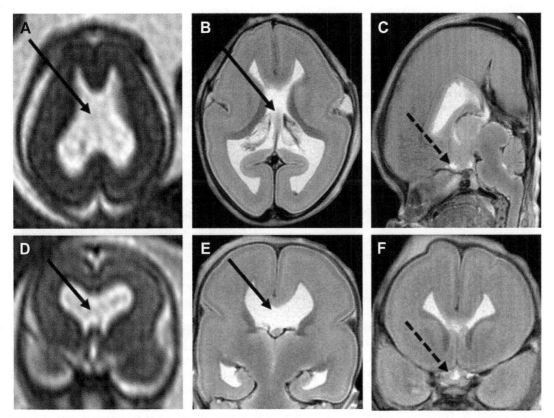

Fig. 9. (*A, D*) Fetal MR imaging at 22 gestational weeks; axial and coronal SSFSE T2-weighted images show (*arrow*) the absence of septum pellucidum. (*B, E*) MR imaging autopsy at 23 gestational weeks confirms (*arrows*) the absence of septum pellucidum. (*C, F*) MR imaging autopsy at 23 gestational weeks; sagittal and coronal TSE T2-weighted images show (*dotted arrows*) hypoplasia of the optic chiasm.

REFERENCES

1. Stiles J, Jernigan TL. The basics of brain development. Neuropsychol Rev 2010;20:327–48.
2. Orioli IM, Castilla EE. Epidemiology of holoprosencephaly: prevalence and risk factors. Am J Med Genet C Semin Med Genet 2010;154C:13–21.
3. Barr M Jr, Hanson JW, Currey K, et al. Holoprosencephaly in infants of diabetic mothers. J Pediatr 1983;102:565–8.
4. Johnson CY, Rasmussen SA. Non-genetic risk factors for holoprosencephaly. Am J Med Genet C Semin Med Genet 2010;154C:73–85.
5. Edison R, Muenke M. The interplay of genetic and environmental factors in craniofacial morphogenesis: holoprosencephaly and the role of cholesterol. Congenit Anom (Kyoto) 2003;43:1–21.
6. Olsen CL, Hughes JP, Youngblood LG, et al. Epidemiology of holoprosencephaly and phenotypic characteristics of affected children: New York State, 1984-1989. Am J Med Genet 1997;73:217–26.
7. Solomon BD, Gropman A, Muenke M. Holoprosencephaly overview. In: Adam MP, Ardinger HH, Pagon RA, et al, editors. GeneReviews® [Internet]. Seattle (WA): University of Washington, Seattle; 1993–2019.
8. Brown SA, Warburton D, Brown LY, et al. Holoprosencephaly due to mutations in ZIC2, a homologue of Drosophila odd-paired. Nat Genet 1998;20: 180–3.
9. Dubourg C, Bendavid C, Pasquier L, et al. Holoprosencephaly. Orphanet J Rare Dis 2007;2:8.
10. Simonis N, Migeotte I, Lambert N, et al. FGFR1 mutations cause Hartsfield syndrome, the unique association of holoprosencephaly and ectrodactyly. J Med Genet 2013;50:585–92.
11. Weaver DD, Solomon BD, Akin-Samson K, et al. Cyclopia (synophthalmia) in Smith-Lemli-Opitz syndrome: first reported case and consideration of mechanism. Am J Med Genet C Semin Med Genet 2010;154C:142–5.
12. Martínez-Frías ML, Bermejo E, Garcia A, et al. Holoprosencephaly associated with caudal dysgenesis: a clinical-epidemiological analysis. Am J Med Genet 1994;53:46–51.
13. DeMyer W, Zeman W. Alobar holoprosencephaly (arhinencephaly) with median cleft lip and palate: clinical, electroencephalographic and nosologic considerations. Confin Neurol 1963;23:1–36.
14. Barkovich AJ, Simon EM, Clegg NJ, et al. Analysis of the cerebral cortex in holoprosencephaly with attention to the sylvian fissures. AJNR Am J Neuroradiol 2002;23(1):143–50.
15. Sepulveda W, Dezerega V, Be C. First-trimester sonographic diagnosis of holoprosencephaly: value of the "butterfly" sign. J Ultrasound Med 2004;23(6): 761–5 [quiz: 766–7].
16. Griffiths PD, Jarvis D. In utero MR imaging of fetal holoprosencephaly: a structured approach to diagnosis and classification. AJNR Am J Neuroradiol 2016;37(3):536–43.
17. Hahn JS, Barnes PD. Neuroimaging advances in holoprosencephaly: refining the spectrum of the midline malformation. Am J Med Genet C Semin Med Genet 2010;154C(1):120–32.
18. Paladini D, Volpe P. Ultrasound of congenital fetal anomalies. London: CRC Press; 2014.
19. Kathuria S, Gregg L, Chen J, et al. Normal cerebral arterial development and variations. Semin Ultrasound CT MR 2011;32(3):242–51.
20. Golden JA. Towards a greater understanding of the pathogenesis of holoprosencephaly. Brain Dev 1999;21(8):513–21.
21. Marcorelles P, Laquerriere A. Neuropathology of holoprosencephaly. Am J Med Genet C Semin Med Genet 2010;154C(1):109–19.
22. Fonda C, Manganaro L, Triulzi FM, et al. RM fetale. Chapter 14. Springer; 2013. p. 131–5.
23. Winter TC, Kennedy AM, Byrne J, et al. The cavum septi pellucidi: why is it important? J Ultrasound Med 2010;29(3):427–44.
24. Winter TC, Kennedy AM, Woodward PJ. Holoprosencephaly: a survey of the entity, with embryology and fetal imaging. Radiographics 2015;35(1):275–90.
25. Silver J, Edwards MA, Levitt P. Immunocytochemical demonstration of early appearing astroglial structures that form boundaries and pathways along axon tracts in the fetal brain. J Comp Neurol 1993; 328:415–36.
26. Gobius I, Morcom L, Suárez R, et al. Astroglial-mediated remodeling of the interhemispheric midline is required for the formation of the corpus callosum. Cell Rep 2016;17(3):735–47.
27. Gobius I, Suárez R, Morcom L. Astroglial-mediated remodeling of the interhemispheric midline during telencephalic development is exclusive to eutherian mammals. Neural Dev 2017;12(1):9.
28. Kanekar S, Shively A, Kaneda H. Malformations of ventral induction. Semin Ultrasound CT MR 2011; 32(3):200–10.
29. Deer E, Nelson C, Moore K, et al. OP14.04: fused fornices CNS findings and outcome in 30 fetal cases. Ultrasound Obstet Gynecol 2011;38(suppl 1):95.
30. Barkovich AJ, Quint DJ. Middle interhemispheric fusion: an unusual variant of holoprosencephaly. AJNR Am J Neuroradiol 1993;14:431–40.
31. Simon EM, Barkovich AJ. Holoprosencephaly: new concepts. Magn Reson Imaging Clin N Am 2001; 9(1):149–64, viii–ix.
32. Pulitzer SB, Simon EM, Crombleholme TM, et al. Prenatal MR findings of the middle interhemispheric variant of holoprosencephaly. AJNR Am J Neuroradiol 2004;25(6):1034–6.

33. De Morsier G. Agénésie du septum lucidum avec mal-formation du tractus optique. La dysplasie septo-optique. Schweiz Arch Neurol Psychiatr 1956;77:267–92.

34. Severino M, Allegri AE, Pistorio A. Midbrain-hindbrain involvement in septo-optic dysplasia. AJNR Am J Neuroradiol 2014;35(8):1586–92.

35. Webb EA, Dattani MT. Septo-optic dysplasia. Eur J Hum Genet 2010;18:393–7.

36. Morishima A, Aranoff GS. Syndrome of septo-optic-pituitary dysplasia: the clinical spectrum. Brain Dev 1986;8:233–9.

37. Raivio T, Avbelj M, McCabe MJ, et al. Genetic overlap in Kallmann syndrome, combined pituitary hormone deficiency, and septo-optic dysplasia. J Clin Endocrinol Metab 2012;97:694–9.

38. Alt C, Shevell MI, Poulin C. Clinical and radiologic spectrum of septo-optic dysplasia: review of 17 cases. J Child Neurol 2017;32(9):797–803.

39. Maurya VK, Ravikumar R, Bhatia M. Septo-optic dysplasia: magnetic resonance imaging findings. Med J Armed Forces India 2015;71(3):287–9.

40. Barkovich AJ, Fram EK, Norman D. Septo-optic dysplasia: MR imaging. Radiology 1989;171(1):189–92.

Diffusion Tensor Imaging of Brain Malformations
Exploring the Internal Architecture

Avner Meoded, MD[a,*], Thierry A.G.M. Huisman, MD[b]

KEYWORDS

- Children • Brain • Malformations • Magnetic resonance imaging • Diffusion tensor imaging
- Fiber tractography

KEY POINTS

- Diffusion tensor imaging (DTI) is an advanced magnetic resonance technique that provides qualitative and quantitative information about the internal architecture of white matter tracts.
- DTI may yield important information about the white matter microstructure in brain malformations that may go underrecognized or not optimally characterized by conventional neuroimaging.
- DTI may better classify various brain malformations that may look similar on conventional/anatomic MR imaging, but may be caused by different pathomechanisms.

INTRODUCTION

Diffusion tensor imaging (DTI) is currently the only MR imaging technique that provides in vivo, noninvasive qualitative and quantitative information about the white matter microarchitecture. DTI and fiber tractography (FT) may provide information that is helpful to better understand the pathogenesis of selected brain malformations. Neuroimaging plays a key role in the diagnostic work-up of brain malformations.[1–3] DTI has shown to provide detailed qualitative and quantitative information in children with brain malformations.[4]

In this review article, we discuss principles of DTI and FT and describe the application of DTI and FT to brain malformations focusing on the added value that DTI and FT may provide compared with conventional neuroimaging.

PRINCIPLES OF DIFFUSION TENSOR IMAGING AND FIBER TRACTOGRAPHY

Diffusion weighted MR imaging generates image contrast based on differences in the mobility of water molecules within tissue.[5]

DTI allows to study the three-dimensional shape and direction of diffusion by adding/sampling diffusion gradients along multiple collinear directions in space. By measuring the complete tensor of the diffusion, the degree of anisotropic diffusion is calculated (fractional anisotropy [FA]).[6–8] Finally, by combining the magnitude and directional information of anisotropic diffusion within the sampled voxels, white matter tracts are calculated/reconstructed by FT (Fig. 1).[9–12]

Diffusion Tensor Imaging and Fiber Tractography of Infratentorial Brain Malformations

Chiari II malformation

Chiari type II malformation (CII) is a complex congenital anomaly of the mid-hindbrain and cervical spinal cord, which occurs in children with non-skin-covered spinal dysraphias/myelomeningoceles.[13,14] Neurologic symptoms are related to the spinal cord dysraphia and cerebral malformation and include abnormal motor function of the lower limbs and impaired ambulation, macrocephaly and signs of increased intracranial pressure

[a] Johns Hopkins All Children's Hospital, 501 6th Avenue South, St Petersburg, FL 33701, USA; [b] Edward B. Singleton Department of Radiology, Texas Children's Hospital, 6701 Fannin Street, Suite 470, Houston, TX 77030, USA
* Corresponding author.
E-mail address: ameoded1@jhmi.edu

Neuroimag Clin N Am 29 (2019) 423–434
https://doi.org/10.1016/j.nic.2019.03.004

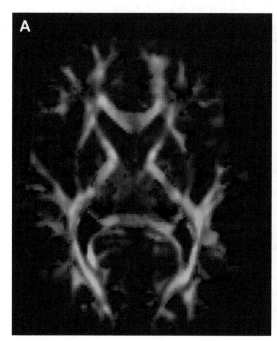
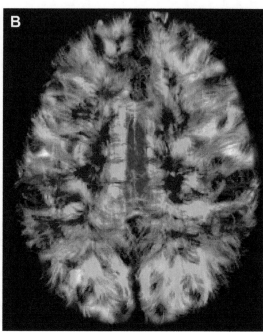

Fig. 1. Axial directionally encoded color (DEC) map (*A*) and whole-brain FT (*B*) of healthy subject. DEC map shows the predominant direction of diffusion, with left to right diffusion in the corpus callosum (*red*), superior-inferior diffusion in the internal capsule (*blue*), and anteroposterior diffusion in the frontal white matter (*green*). Whole-brain tractography (*B*) is a three-dimensional representation of white matter fibers.

caused by hydrocephalus. In addition, cranial nerve palsy, nystagmus, sleep apnea, and dysphagia may be observed.[15]

A small posterior fossa is the key neuroimaging finding of CII. In addition, cerebellar hypoplasia, downward and upward herniation of the cerebellar vermis, wrapping of the cerebellar hemispheres around the brainstem, pontine hypoplasia, tectal beaking, kinking of the medulla, and widening of the foramen magnum may be seen in the posterior fossa.[14] Hydrocephalus is usually the main neuroimaging finding involving the supratentorial brain in CII. Additional classic supratentorial neuroimaging findings include abnormalities of the corpus callosum and hippocampal commissure, low-position of the anterior commissure, a prominent interthalamic adhesion (massa intermedia), and gray matter heterotopia.[16]

Analysis of the infratentorial and supratentorial white matter with DTI in patients with CII has been reported. Quantitative DTI allowed to analyze DTI scalars along several white matter tracts, such as in the corpus callosum, inferior longitudinal fasciculus, posterior corona radiata, anterior limb of the internal capsule, cerebral peduncles, and cingulum in children with CII compared with control subjects.[17–21] DTI changes suggest an underlying abnormal development with impaired myelination and secondary injury of the white matter tracts for

example, because of high-grade hydrocephalus in CII.[18,21] Within the posterior fossa, qualitative evaluation of DTI and FT data in CII revealed a more vertical orientation of the middle cerebellar peduncle and a reduction in size of all cerebellar peduncles and transverse pontine fibers (TPF) (**Figs. 2** and **3**).[4] A decrease in size of the TPF is the most likely explanation of pontine hypoplasia that is usually seen in CII. In addition, our group previously showed an anterior displacement of the dentate nuclei.[4] This is most likely caused by the wrapping of the brainstem by the cerebellar hemispheres with anterior displacement of the deep cerebellar nuclei. Quantitative evaluation of the cerebellar white matter tracts in CII showed reduction in FA of the MCPs.[22] The most likely explanation is a decrease in fiber density caused by cerebellar hypoplasia. Recently, quantitative analysis of fetal DTI data showed a significant increase in FA in the midbrain of fetuses with CII compared with normal developing fetuses.[23] Extrinsic compression of the fetal brainstem in the axial plane leading to impaired diffusion of water molecules in the axial plane, but not in the craniocaudal direction, has been suggested and seems to be the most likely explanation for this finding. The measurement of FA within the midbrain may help to differentiate fetuses with skin-covered and non-skin-covered spinal dysraphia.

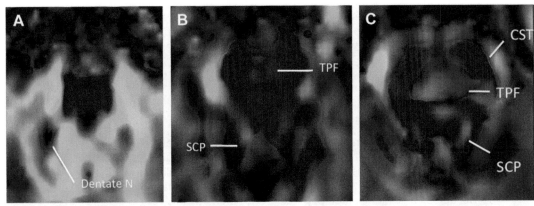

Fig. 2. A child with CII. (*A–C*) Axial DEC maps reveal anteromedial displacement of the dentate nuclei and more vertical orientation of the MCPs. CST, corticospinal tract; SCP, superior cerebellar peduncle. (*Adapted from* Chokshi FH, Poretti A, Meoded A, et al. Normal and abnormal development of the cerebellum and brainstem as depicted by diffusion tensor imaging. *Seminars in Ultrasound, CT, and MR* 2011;32:539-554; with permission.)

Joubert syndrome

Joubert syndrome (JS) is an autosomal-recessive mid-hindbrain malformation caused by mutations in more than 30 genes that encode for proteins of the nonmotile primary cilia.[24] Children with JS present with hypotonia, cerebellar ataxia, ocular motor apraxia, neonatal breathing dysregulation, and intellectual disability of variable severity.

The "molar tooth sign" is the diagnostic MR imaging criterion for JS and consists of elongated, thickened, and horizontally oriented superior cerebellar peduncle (SCPs) and a deep interpeduncular fossa, best seen on axial imaging.[25] In addition, hypoplasia and dysplasia of the remaining cerebellar vermis is a consistent finding in JS. In JS, the spectrum of neuroimaging findings goes beyond the molar tooth sign and hypodysplasia of the cerebellar vermis.[26] Morphologic abnormalities of the brainstem are present in about

30% of patients and include a dysmorphic tectum and midbrain, thickening and elongation of the midbrain, and a small pons. Supratentorial involvement occurs in about 30% of patients and includes callosal dysgenesis, cephaloceles, hippocampal malrotation, migrational disorders, and ventriculomegaly and occasional hypothalamic hamartomas.

In JS, directionally encoded color (DEC) maps show the horizontal orientation of the SCP (completely green color coded) compared with the normal slight vertical orientation (green-blue color coded) (**Fig. 4**).[27–29] In addition, DTI may reveal an abnormal, more lateral location of the deep cerebellar nuclei.[28,29] Moreover, DTI and FT reveal absence of decussation of both the SCPs (missing red dot adjacent to the deep interpeduncular fossa) and corticospinal tract (CSTs) (see **Fig. 4**).[28,29] Absence of SCPs and CSTs

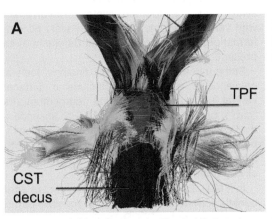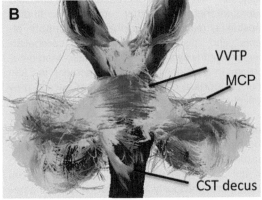

Fig. 3. Same child with CII as in Fig. 2. (*A*) Anterior projection of FT shows moderate decrease of the TPF and decreased density of CST decussating fibers. (*B*) Normal subject for comparison. VVTP, ventro-ventral transverse pontine fibers. (*Adapted from* Chokshi FH, Poretti A, Meoded A, et al. Normal and abnormal development of the cerebellum and brainstem as depicted by diffusion tensor imaging. *Seminars in Ultrasound, CT, and MR* 2011;32:539-554; with permission.)

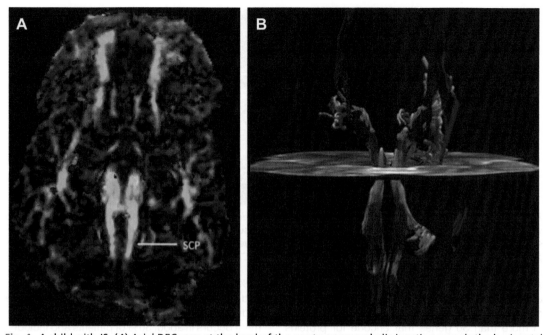

Fig. 4. A child with JS. (*A*) Axial DEC map at the level of the pontomesencephalic junction reveals the horizontal orientation of the SCPs (*green color, arrows*) and the absence of the *red dot* within the midbrain representing the failure of SCPs to decussate. (*B*) Coronal projection of FT superimposed on an axial T2-weighted image shows the course of the CSTs without identifiable crossing fibers (*horizontal red fibers*) at the level of the lower medulla. A group of noncrossing fibers of the SCPs is also displayed on the left side (*green encoded*). (*Adapted from* Poretti A, Boltshauser E, Loenneker T, et al. Diffusion tensor imaging in Joubert syndrome. *AJNR Am J Neuroradiol* 2007;28:1929-1933; with permission.)

decussation in JS has been previously shown by neuropathology.[30,31] JS is now considered an axonal guidance disorder secondary to the malfunction of the nonmotile cilia.[32] Recently, DTI showed thinning of the dorsal TPF and MCPs in two patients with JS.[33] Furthermore, our group performed atlas-based analysis of the entire brain in one child with JS and five age-matched control subjects.[34] We found a decrease in FA in selected supratentorial white matter regions. This finding most likely results from trophic trans-synaptic effects and disconnection of the cerebellar-cerebral pathway secondary to a malformed cerebellum. In addition, we found an increase in FA in multiple cortical gray matter regions, which may reflect disrupted cortical neuronal radial glial cell scaffolding and neuronal laminar organization as reported in mice with *Arl13b* mutations, one of the genes associated with JS.[35] Finally, mostly based on DTI findings (absence of decussation of the SCPs and elongated, horizontal [green] SCPs), we previously suggested that tectocerebellar dysraphism with occipital encephalocele may not be a distinct disorder, but represents the structural representation of a heterogeneous group of disorders belonging to the spectrum of JS (**Fig. 5**).[26]

Pontine tegmental cap dysplasia

Pontine tegmental cap dysplasis (PTCD) is a rare sporadic brainstem malformation with unknown genotype and no familial recurrence. Children with PTCD present with involvement of vestibulo-cochlear, facial, trigeminal, and glossopharyngeal nerves, resulting in hearing loss, facial paralysis, trigeminal anesthesia, and difficulty in swallowing.[36] In addition, systemic involvement with vertebral segmentation anomalies, rib malformations, and congenital heart defects may be present.

Pathognomonic morphologic findings seen on conventional neuroimaging include a flattened ventral pons, vaulted pontine tegmentum (the "cap"), partial absence of the MCPs, absence of the inferior cerebellar peduncle (ICPs), vermian hypoplasia, a molar tooth–like aspect of the ponto-mesencephalic junction, and absent inferior olivary prominence.[36,37]

In PTCD, DTI and FT revealed significant additional information regarding the possible pathogenesis. To date, PTCD is also considered to be an axonal guidance disorder.[32] Axial DEC maps do not show the TPF at the level of the pons likely explaining the flattened pons (**Figs. 6** and **7**).[37,38] However, DEC maps

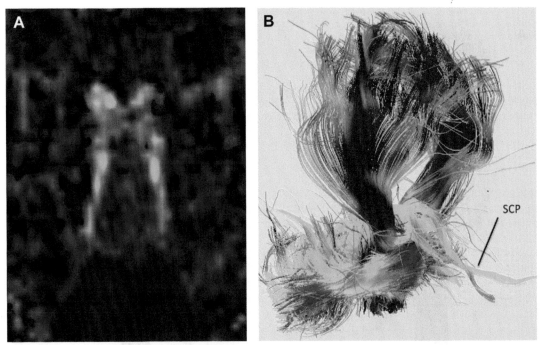

Fig. 5. A 4-year-old patient with tecto-cerebellar dysraphism with occipital meningo-encephalocele. Axial DEC map at the level of (A) pontomesencephalic region and (B) an anterolateral projection of a matching region fiber tractography. The SCPs are elongated and horizontal showing a molar tooth–like form. The absence of the midline *red dot* at the level of the pontomesencephalic junction suggests the absence of the decussation of the SCP. Moreover, the SCPs have an aberrant horizontal projection anteriorly to the brainstem. All other white matter tracts appear normal. (*Adapted from* Chokshi FH, Poretti A, Meoded A, et al. Normal and abnormal development of the cerebellum and brainstem as depicted by diffusion tensor imaging. *Seminars in Ultrasound, CT, and MR* 2011;32:539-554; with permission.)

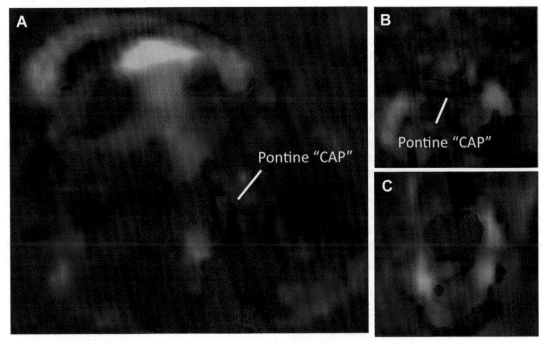

Fig. 6. A child with PTCD. (A) Midsagittal and (B, C) axial DEC maps reveal the absence of TPF in the ventral and middle pons and an ectopic band of fibers (horizontal orientation) dorsal to the pons. (*From* Chokshi FH, Poretti A, Meoded A, et al. Normal and abnormal development of the cerebellum and brainstem as depicted by diffusion tensor imaging. Semin Ultrasound CT MR 2011;32:539–54; with permission.)

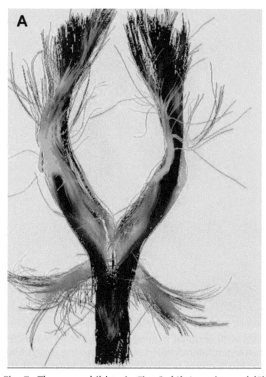

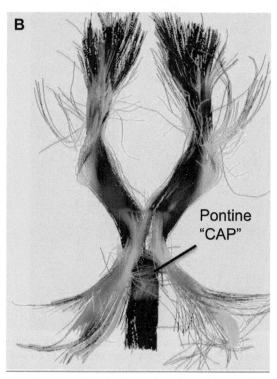

Fig. 7. The same child as in Fig. 6. (*A*) Anterior and (*B*) posterior coronal projections of FT show absence of TPF and presence of an ectopic band of fibers dorsal to the pons (*arrow* in *B*). (*From* Chokshi FH, Poretti A, Meoded A, et al. Normal and abnormal development of the cerebellum and brainstem as depicted by diffusion tensor imaging. Semin Ultrasound CT MR 2011;32:539–54; with permission.)

revealed in all patients an abnormal bundle of transversely oriented fibers (red) that cross the midline along the dorsal pons and extend between both MCPs to form the pontine tegmental cap. It is unclear whether these fibers are continuous with the MCP or not. Recently, a study using HARDI data in PTCD revealed the presence of misoriented fibers connecting the base of the pons with the cerebellar hemispheres through the MCPs (peripontine arcuate fibers), some of which seemed to join the dorsal ectopic band.[39] In addition, DEC maps also confirmed the hypoplasia of the MCPs, absence of the ICPs, and mild elongation and lateral displacement of the SCPs resulting in a molar tooth–like appearance. Finally, the midline red dot at the pontomesencephalic junction is typically not present suggesting lack of SCPs decussation.[37,38]

Horizontal gaze palsy with progressive scoliosis

Horizontal gaze palsy with progressive scoliosis (HGPPS) is a rare autosomal-recessive disorder caused by mutations in *ROBO3*, which encodes a receptor required for axonal guidance.[40] Children with HGPPS present with congenital absence of horizontal eye movements, preservation of vertical gaze and convergence, and progressive

development of scoliosis in childhood.[41] Neurocognitive functions are typically preserved.

Neuroimaging findings are pathognomonic and include a butterfly-shaped medulla caused by the missing prominence of the gracile and cuneate nuclei, and prominent inferior olivary nuclei with respect to the medullary pyramids.[42] In addition, the pons is hypoplastic and has a dorsal midline cleft with absence of the bulging contour of facial colliculi.[42]

In HGPPS, DTI and FT show a complete ipsilateral course of the CSTs without decussation at the level of the lower medulla.[43,44] The sensorimotor tracts revealed only ipsilateral ascending fibers.[43] The uncrossed ascending course of the sensory tracts may result in lack of bilateral integration of proprioceptive stimuli and be responsible for the development of scoliosis. The decussation of the SCPs at the level of the pontomesencephalic junction could not be identified (absent midline red dot).[43–45]

Diffusion Tensor Imaging and Fiber Tractography of Supratentorial Brain Malformations

Agenesis of the corpus callosum

The corpus callosum is the largest and best visualized cerebral commissure. It is composed of five sections: (1) rostrum, (2) genu, (3) body (forming the frontal segment), (4) isthmus (sensory-motor), and (5) splenium (parieto-occipital).[46] The corpus callosum may be completely absent (agenesis) or partially formed (hypogenesis). Additionally, malformations of the other commissures (anterior and hippocampal commissures) may be associated with corpus callosum agenesis or hypogenesis leading to a complex spectrum of various commissural disorders.[46] Moreover, in addition to anomalies of the other telencephalic commissures, anomalies of the corpus callosum are often associated with additional cerebral or cerebellar abnormalities, such as interhemispheric cysts, malformations of the cortical development, cerebellar dysgenesis, cephaloceles, or hypothalamic anomalies.[47–49]

Callosal anomalies may be isolated or be part of many complex syndromes, such as Aicardi syndrome, fetal alcohol syndrome, CII malformation, Dandy-Walker malformation, nonketotic hyperglycinemia, or pyruvate dehydrogenase deficiency. The most frequent is probably Aicardi syndrome, a likely X-linked dominant disorder characterized by the triad of callosal agenesis, infantile spasms, and chorioretinal lacunae.[50]

DTI and FT have focused on several anatomic features of agenesis and dysgenesis of the corpus callosum, allowing better understanding of their development during the prenatal and postnatal periods.[4,51]

In patients with agenesis of the corpus callosum, next to the lack of the left-right crossing commissural fibers, the most obvious DTI finding is the presence of the bilateral bundles of Probst as large, anteroposterior oriented (green on color-coded FA maps), intrahemispheric, heterotopic white matter tracts that are coursing along the medial and superior wall of the lateral ventricles (Fig. 8). The bundles of Probst are formed from misdirected callosal axons and may be depicted also in fetuses using DTI (Fig. 9).[4]

Holoprosencephaly

Holoprosencephaly (HPE) is a complex human brain malformation caused by incomplete cleavage of the telencephalon and absent or poor development of the midline structures.[52,53] This embryologic process is normally complete by the fifth week of gestation. The cause of HPE is heterogeneous and includes environmental and multiple chromosomal and genetic causes.

HPE has traditionally been classified into three grades of increasing severity based on the major neuroanatomic findings: (1) lobar HPE, where the cerebral hemispheres are rather well-developed and separated (including thalamic nuclei) with rudimentary formation of the frontal horns of the lateral ventricles and nonseparation only of the most rostral/ventral parts of the striatum and neocortex with absence of the corpus callosum in the affected region; (2) semilobar HPE with lack of separation of the anterior part of the hemispheres and incomplete separation of the deep gray matter nuclei, but separation of the posterior and inferior parts of the hemispheres resulting in presence of the posterior horns and trigones of the lateral ventricles and of the splenium of the corpus callosum; and (3) alobar

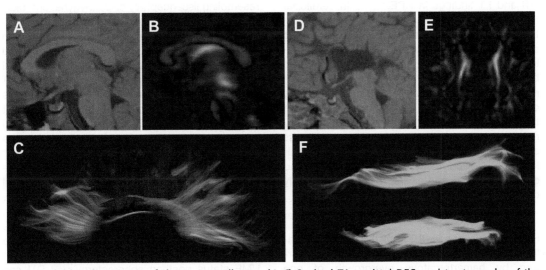

Fig. 8. A child with agenesis of the corpus callosum. (A–C) Sagittal T1, sagittal DEC, and tractography of the normal corpus callosum. (D–F) Corresponding images of a patient with corpus callosum agenesis. The bundles of Probst are noted as large, anteroposterior-oriented (green on DEC maps) white matter tracts that are running along the medial and superior wall of the lateral ventricles.

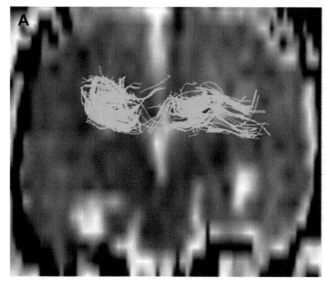
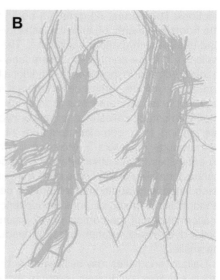

Fig. 9. Images in a fetus with corpus callosum agenesis at 34 6/7 weeks of gestation. (*A*) FT superimposed on a coronal T2-weighted HASTE image shows the Probst bundles as thick, green parallel bundles coursing medially to the lateral ventricles. No callosal fibers are noted crossing the midline. (*B*) Three-dimensional tractography reconstruction of the Probst bundles. (*From* Meoded A, Poretti A, Tekes A, et al. Prenatal MR diffusion tractography in a fetus with complete corpus callosum agenesis. *Neuropediatrics* 2011; 42:122–123; with permission.)

HPE, the most severe form with a complete or nearly complete lack of separation of the cerebral hemispheres, including basal ganglia, thalami and hypothalamic nuclei, a single midline forebrain ventricle (holoventricle), which often communicates with a dorsal cyst, and a complete absence of the interhemispheric fissure, falx cerebri, and corpus callosum.[54,55]

We are aware of only a few articles reporting DTI and FT findings in HPE.[4,56–59] In semilobar HPE, DTI and fiber tracking revealed white matter structures not apparent on routine imaging sequences, which are in agreement with pathologic descriptions of the holoprosencephalic brain.[57] In one of our unpublished cases we noted the fused caudates as previously described by Rollins.[57] In addition, we noticed the prominent anterior commissure most likely reflecting reorganization mechanism as a results of the abnormal formation of the corpus callosum (Fig. 10). Finally, aberrant brainstem and cerebellar white matter tracts were previously described in alobar HPE.[59]

Hemimegalencephaly

Hemimegalencephaly (HME), or unilateral megalencephaly, is an uncommon condition characterized by hamartomatous overgrowth of one cerebral hemisphere. Its pathogenesis is poorly understood. HME has been proposed to result from an early primary disorder of neuroepithelial lineage and cellular growth with secondary migratory disturbance.[60] Affected children present during the first days or weeks of life with medically intractable seizures, global developmental delay, and cognitive impairment.[61]

Conventional neuroimaging shows typically an asymmetric enlargement of the affected hemisphere with an abnormal gyral pattern including broad gyri, shallow sulci and cortical thickening resembling lissencephaly or pachygyria, and blurring of the cortical–white matter junction.[4] The ipsilateral ventricle appears typically enlarged with straightening of the frontal horn and/or unilateral colpocephaly. The white matter shows abnormal high T2 signal intensity because of absent or incomplete myelination.[62] The corpus callosum is almost always asymmetrical with enlargement and dysplasia of the affected side.[63] Additional infratentorial size asymmetry may be noted in a smaller proportion of cases.

DTI may show a complete disorganization of the ipsilateral white matter fibers with an abnormal concentric orientation around the ventricle. Abnormal interhemispheric fibers and asymmetric thickening of ipsilateral white matter tracts have been described in HME.[64,65] Finally, DTI can add valuable information in patients affected with HME status posthemispherectomy.[26,66] DTI can enhance the understanding of the structural cerebral plasticity in patients after hemispherectomy (Fig. 11).

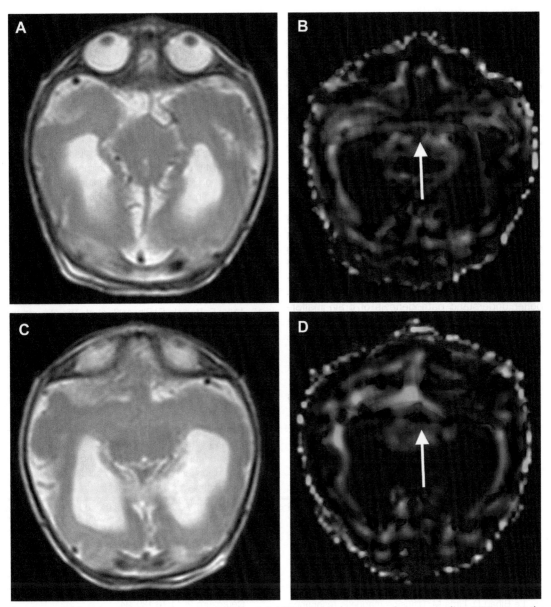

Fig. 10. A child with semilobar holoprosencephaly. Axial T2-weighted image and corresponding DEC map at the level of the anterior commissure (*A, B*) and the caudates (*C, D*) demonstrate failure of cleavage of the frontal and parietal lobes with holoventricle extending over the midline. Prominent anterior commissure (*arrow* in *B*) and fused caudate nuclei (*arrow* in *D*) are noted.

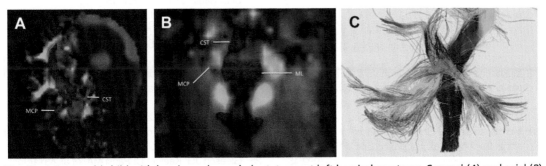

Fig. 11. A 3-year-old child with hemimegalencephaly status post left hemispherectomy. Coronal (*A*) and axial (*B*) DEC maps and posterior projection of FT (*C*). The size of the ipsilesional CST is significant, the size of the contralesional MCP is slightly reduced. The size of the medial lemniscus within the brainstem is symmetric. (*Adapted from* Chokshi FH, Poretti A, Meoded A, et al. Normal and abnormal development of the cerebellum and brainstem as depicted by diffusion tensor imaging. *Seminars in Ultrasound, CT, and MR* 2011;32:539-554; with permission.)

SUMMARY

DTI and FT provide in vivo, noninvasive detailed qualitative and quantitative information about white matter microstructural integrity and (dys)-organization in children with brain malformations. In addition, the normal and abnormal connectivity between different anatomic centers within the brain can be evaluated. Moreover, the combination of DTI and FT findings in humans with genetic analyses in animal models might suggest the involvement of particular genes in selected malformations. Finally, in the future the correlation of quantitative DTI findings in specific white matter regions with measurements of cognitive functions might be a follow-up biomarker for cognitive and behavioral therapies in children with brain malformations. All this information may be helpful to better understand pathogenesis of brain malformations and possibly predict cognitive outcome for children with brain malformations.

REFERENCES

1. Doherty D, Millen KJ, Barkovich AJ. Midbrain and hindbrain malformations: advances in clinical diagnosis, imaging, and genetics. Lancet Neurol 2013; 12:381–93.

2. Bosemani T, Orman G, Boltshauser E, et al. Congenital abnormalities of the posterior fossa. Radiographics 2015;35:200–20.

3. Jissendi-Tchofo P, Severino M, Nguema-Edzang B, et al. Update on neuroimaging phenotypes of mid-hindbrain malformations. Neuroradiology 2015;57: 113–38.

4. Poretti A, Meoded A, Rossi A, et al. Diffusion tensor imaging and fiber tractography in brain malformations. Pediatr Radiol 2013;43:28–54.

5. Le Bihan D, Lima M. Diffusion magnetic resonance imaging: what water tells us about biological tissues. PLoS Biol 2015;13:e1002203.

6. Basser PJ, Jones DK. Diffusion-tensor MRI: theory, experimental design and data analysis: a technical review. NMR Biomed 2002;15:456–67.

7. Ito R, Mori S, Melhem ER. Diffusion tensor brain imaging and tractography. Neuroimaging Clin N Am 2002;12:1–19.

8. Mukherjee P, Berman JI, Chung SW, et al. Diffusion tensor MR imaging and fiber tractography: theoretic underpinnings. AJNR Am J Neuroradiol 2008;29: 632–41.

9. Mori S, Crain BJ, Chacko VP, et al. Three-dimensional tracking of axonal projections in the brain by magnetic resonance imaging. Ann Neurol 1999;45: 265–9.

10. Ciccarelli O, Catani M, Johansen-Berg H, et al. Diffusion-based tractography in neurological disorders: concepts, applications, and future developments. Lancet Neurol 2008;7:715–27.

11. Chung HW, Chou MC, Chen CY. Principles and limitations of computational algorithms in clinical diffusion tensor MR tractography. AJNR Am J Neuroradiol 2011;32:3–13.

12. Huisman TA, Bosemani T, Poretti A. Diffusion tensor imaging for brain malformations: does it help? Neuroimaging Clin N Am 2014;24:619–37.

13. McLone DG, Dias MS. The Chiari II malformation: cause and impact. Childs Nerv Syst 2003;19: 540–50.

14. Juranek J, Salman MS. Anomalous development of brain structure and function in spina bifida myelomeningocele. Dev Disabil Res Rev 2010; 16:23–30.

15. Stevenson KL. Chiari type II malformation: past, present, and future. Neurosurg Focus 2004;16:E5.

16. Miller E, Widjaja E, Blaser S, et al. The old and the new: supratentorial MR findings in Chiari II malformation. Childs Nerv Syst 2008;24:563–75.

17. Vachha B, Adams RC, Rollins NK. Limbic tract anomalies in pediatric myelomeningocele and Chiari II malformation: anatomic correlations with memory and learning: initial investigation. Radiology 2006; 240:194–202.

18. Hasan KM, Eluvathingal TJ, Kramer LA, et al. White matter microstructural abnormalities in children with spina bifida myelomeningocele and hydrocephalus: a diffusion tensor tractography study of the association pathways. J Magn Reson Imaging 2008;27: 700–9.

19. Herweh C, Akbar M, Wengenroth M, et al. DTI of commissural fibers in patients with Chiari II-malformation. Neuroimage 2009;44:306–11.

20. Kumar M, Rathore RK, Srivastava A, et al. Correlation of diffusion tensor imaging metrics with neurocognitive function in Chiari I malformation. World Neurosurg 2011;76:189–94.

21. Ou X, Glasier CM, Snow JH. Diffusion tensor imaging evaluation of white matter in adolescents with myelomeningocele and Chiari II malformation. Pediatr Radiol 2011;41:1407–15.

22. Herweh C, Akbar M, Wengenroth M, et al. Reduced anisotropy in the middle cerebellar peduncle in Chiari-II malformation. Cerebellum 2010;9:303–9.

23. Woitek R, Prayer D, Weber M, et al. Fetal diffusion tensor quantification of brainstem pathology in Chiari II malformation. Eur Radiol 2016;26(5): 1274–83.

24. Romani M, Micalizzi A, Valente EM. Joubert syndrome: congenital cerebellar ataxia with the molar tooth. Lancet Neurol 2013;12:894–905.

25. Gleeson JG, Keeler LC, Parisi MA, et al. Molar tooth sign of the midbrain-hindbrain junction: occurrence in multiple distinct syndromes. Am J Med Genet A 2004;125:125–34 [discussion: 117].

26. Chokshi FH, Poretti A, Meoded A, et al. Normal and abnormal development of the cerebellum and brainstem as depicted by diffusion tensor imaging. Semin Ultrasound CT MR 2011;32:539–54.

27. Lee SK, Kim DI, Kim J, et al. Diffusion-tensor MR imaging and fiber tractography: a new method of describing aberrant fiber connections in developmental CNS anomalies. Radiographics 2005;25:53–65 [discussion: 66–8].

28. Widjaja E, Blaser S, Raybaud C. Diffusion tensor imaging of midline posterior fossa malformations. Pediatr Radiol 2006;36:510–7.

29. Poretti A, Boltshauser E, Loenneker T, et al. Diffusion tensor imaging in Joubert syndrome. AJNR Am J Neuroradiol 2007;28:1929–33.

30. Friede RL, Boltshauser E. Uncommon syndromes of cerebellar vermis aplasia. I: Joubert syndrome. Dev Med Child Neurol 1978;20:758–63.

31. Yachnis AT, Rorke LB. Neuropathology of Joubert syndrome. J Child Neurol 1999;14:655–9 [discussion: 669–72].

32. Engle EC. Human genetic disorders of axon guidance. Cold Spring Harb Perspect Biol 2010;2:a001784.

33. Hsu CC, Kwan GN, Bhuta S. High-resolution diffusion tensor imaging and tractography in Joubert syndrome: beyond molar tooth sign. Pediatr Neurol 2015;53:47–52.

34. Bosemani T, Baum J, Meoded A, et al. Impaired growth and abnormal microstructure of supratentorial gray and white matter regions in a child with Joubert syndrome. Neurographics 2015;5(5):209–16.

35. Higginbotham H, Eom TY, Mariani LE, et al. Arl13b in primary cilia regulates the migration and placement of interneurons in the developing cerebral cortex. Dev Cell 2012;23:925–38.

36. Barth PG, Majoie CB, Caan MW, et al. Pontine tegmental cap dysplasia: a novel brain malformation with a defect in axonal guidance. Brain 2007;130:2258–66.

37. Jissendi-Tchofo P, Doherty D, McGillivray G, et al. Pontine tegmental cap dysplasia: MR imaging and diffusion tensor imaging features of impaired axonal navigation. AJNR Am J Neuroradiol 2009;30:113–9.

38. Briguglio M, Pinelli L, Giordano L, et al. Pontine tegmental cap dysplasia: developmental and cognitive outcome in three adolescent patients. Orphanet J Rare Dis 2011;6:36.

39. Caan MW, Barth PG, Niermeijer JM, et al. Ectopic peripontine arcuate fibres, a novel finding in pontine tegmental cap dysplasia. Eur J Paediatr Neurol 2014;18:434–8.

40. Jen JC, Chan WM, Bosley TM, et al. Mutations in a human ROBO gene disrupt hindbrain axon pathway crossing and morphogenesis. Science 2004;304:1509–13.

41. Bosley TM, Salih MA, Jen JC, et al. Neurologic features of horizontal gaze palsy and progressive scoliosis with mutations in ROBO3. Neurology 2005;64:1196–203.

42. Rossi A, Catala M, Biancheri R, et al. MR imaging of brain-stem hypoplasia in horizontal gaze palsy with progressive scoliosis. AJNR Am J Neuroradiol 2004;25:1046–8.

43. Haller S, Wetzel SG, Lutschg J. Functional MRI, DTI and neurophysiology in horizontal gaze palsy with progressive scoliosis. Neuroradiology 2008;50:453–9.

44. Avadhani A, Ilayaraja V, Shetty AP, et al. Diffusion tensor imaging in horizontal gaze palsy with progressive scoliosis. Magn Reson Imaging 2010;28:212–6.

45. Sicotte NL, Salamon G, Shattuck DW, et al. Diffusion tensor MRI shows abnormal brainstem crossing fibers associated with ROBO3 mutations. Neurology 2006;67:519–21.

46. Raybaud C. The corpus callosum, the other great forebrain commissures, and the septum pellucidum: anatomy, development, and malformation. Neuroradiology 2010;52:447–77.

47. Barkovich AJ, Norman D. Anomalies of the corpus callosum: correlation with further anomalies of the brain. AJR Am J Roentgenol 1988;151:171–9.

48. Sztriha L. Spectrum of corpus callosum agenesis. Pediatr Neurol 2005;32:94–101.

49. Hetts SW, Sherr EH, Chao S, et al. Anomalies of the corpus callosum: an MR analysis of the phenotypic spectrum of associated malformations. AJR Am J Roentgenol 2006;187:1343–8.

50. Aicardi J. Aicardi syndrome. Brain Dev 2005;27:164–71.

51. Meoded A, Poretti A, Tekes A, et al. Prenatal MR diffusion tractography in a fetus with complete corpus callosum agenesis. Neuropediatrics 2011;42:122–3.

52. Dubourg C, Bendavid C, Pasquier L, et al. Holoprosencephaly. Orphanet J Rare Dis 2007;2:8.

53. Raam MS, Solomon BD, Muenke M. Holoprosencephaly: a guide to diagnosis and clinical management. Indian Pediatr 2011;48:457–66.

54. Hahn JS, Barnes PD. Neuroimaging advances in holoprosencephaly: refining the spectrum of the midline malformation. Am J Med Genet C Semin Med Genet 2010;154C:120–32.

55. Barkovich AJ, Simon EM, Clegg NJ, et al. Analysis of the cerebral cortex in holoprosencephaly with attention to the sylvian fissures. AJNR Am J Neuroradiol 2002;23:143–50.

56. Bulakbasi N, Cancuri O, Kocaoglu M. The middle interhemispheric variant of holoprosencephaly: magnetic resonance and diffusion tensor imaging findings. Br J Radiol 2016;89:20160115.

57. Rollins N. Semilobar holoprosencephaly seen with diffusion tensor imaging and fiber tracking. AJNR Am J Neuroradiol 2005;26:2148–52.

58. Ortiz B, Herrera DA, Vargas S. Clinical application of diffusion tensor imaging and tractography in a child with holoprosencephaly. Biomedica 2011;31:164–7 [in Spanish].

59. Albayram S, Melhem ER, Mori S, et al. Holoprosencephaly in children: diffusion tensor MR imaging of white matter tracts of the brainstem: initial experience. Radiology 2002;223:645–51.

60. Flores-Sarnat L, Sarnat HB, Davila-Gutierrez G, et al. Hemimegalencephaly: part 2. Neuropathology suggests a disorder of cellular lineage. J Child Neurol 2003;18:776–85.

61. Hung PC, Wang HS. Hemimegalencephaly: cranial sonographic findings in neonates. J Clin Ultrasound 2005;33:243–7.

62. Yagishita A, Arai N, Tamagawa K, et al. Hemimegalencephaly: signal changes suggesting abnormal myelination on MRI. Neuroradiology 1998;40:734–8.

63. Griffiths PD, Welch RJ, Gardner-Medwin D, et al. The radiological features of hemimegalencephaly including three cases associated with proteus syndrome. Neuropediatrics 1994;25:140–4.

64. Sato N, Ota M, Yagishita A, et al. Aberrant midsagittal fiber tracts in patients with hemimegalencephaly. AJNR Am J Neuroradiol 2008;29:823–7.

65. Takahashi T, Sato N, Ota M, et al. Asymmetrical interhemispheric fiber tracts in patients with hemimegalencephaly on diffusion tensor magnetic resonance imaging. J Neuroradiol 2009;36:249–54.

66. Meoded A, Faria AV, Hartman AL, et al. Cerebral reorganization after hemispherectomy: a DTI study. AJNR Am J Neuroradiol 2016;37:924–31.

Connectomics in Brain Malformations
How Is the Malformed Brain Wired?

Avner Meoded, MD[a],*, Thierry A.G.M. Huisman, MD[b]

KEYWORDS

• Diffusion tensor imaging • Structural connectome • Malformations • Brain • Children

KEY POINTS

- The structural connectome is a comprehensive structural description of the network of elements and connections forming the brain.
- In recent years this framework has progressively been used to investigate the pediatric brain during development and in pediatric central nervous system diseases.
- Connectomics provide novel insights into aberrant brain organization in congenital brain malformations.

INTRODUCTION

The term "connectome" embodies the advances of over a century of neuroscientific innovation and reflects the agenda for a new era: the era of the brain networks.[1] The human connectome is the comprehensive structural description of the network of elements and connections forming the human brain and can be mathematically described as a neural graph.[2–4] Brain graphs provide a relatively simple and increasingly popular way of modeling the human brain connectome, using graph theory to abstractly define the brain as a set of anatomic regions, for example, nodes, and structural connections, for example, edges.[4,5]

The main impact of the graph theory is to promote a change of perspective in how we view the brain.[6] The connectome provides a unified, time-invariant and readily available neuroinformatics resource that can be used in virtually all areas of experimental and theoretic neuroscience.[7] Network analyses of brain connectivity have begun to yield important insights into brain organization of humans and nonhuman primates.[8]

Network measures are critical for creating metrics that allow the comparison of connectivity patterns across individuals, imaging modalities, as well as clinical conditions. Graph measures allow the characterization of network structure by identifying local contributions of individual nodes and connections, as well as the network's global capacity to integrate/process information, or its tendency to form interconnected communities or modules.[9] Complex network properties have been identified with some consistency in all modalities of neuroimaging data and over a range of spatial and timescales. Conserved properties include small-worldness, high efficiency of information transfer for low wiring cost, modularity, and the existence of network hubs.[10–12] In recent years this framework has been used to investigate the pediatric brain. Normal brain development is characterized by continuous and significant network evolution throughout infancy, childhood, and adolescence, following specific maturational steps. Uncovering these complicated processes is crucial to understanding the formation of the brain network. With the recent advancement of

[a] Pediatric Radiology and Neuroradiology, Johns Hopkins University School of Medicine, Johns Hopkins All Children's Hospital, 501 Sixth Avenue South, St Petersburg, FL 33701, USA; [b] Edward B. Singleton Department of Radiology, Texas Children's Hospital, 6701 Fannin Street, Suite 470, Houston, TX 77030, USA
* Corresponding author.
E-mail address: ameoded1@jhmi.edu

Neuroimag Clin N Am 29 (2019) 435–444
https://doi.org/10.1016/j.nic.2019.03.005
1052-5149/19/© 2019 Elsevier Inc. All rights reserved.

noninvasive neuroimaging techniques to study the pediatric brain, the comprehensive macroscale connectome can be evaluated in children in vivo.

Currently, various neurodevelopmental disorders, including congenital brain malformations, may be considered as connectopathies or disconnection syndromes, and thus the structural connectome may help us understand the pathogenesis and implication for cognitive and behavioral functions of brain disorders from a network perspective.[13–15]

In this review article, we focus on the up-to-date principles of the pediatric structural connectome and its potential use to study congenital brain malformations.

HOW TO BUILD THE PEDIATRIC STRUCTURAL CONNECTOME

Several important steps are needed for the reconstruction of the structural connectome.[16] The 2 key components required for structural connectome reconstruction are a node and an edge. Nodes correspond to neuronal elements, for example, gray matter voxels or brain regions. For this purpose high-resolution T1-weighted MR imaging is needed. Edges represent measures of structural association between cortical regions and are derived from diffusion tensor imaging (DTI) tractography.

NODES: CORTICAL PARCELLATION

Different parcellations of the human brain exist. Atlases of brain areas generated using anatomic and functional parcellation schemes are available (Fig. 1).[1] In children, the accurate identification of cortical regions at high resolution is challenging because sulci continue to develop after birth resulting in a rapidly changing complexity of the brain surface/sulci. In addition, the MR imaging contrast in the brain of young children varies considerably with age, and it is not always straightforward to delineate what constitutes a normal appearance and what degree of variability reflects a pathologic condition. For pediatric brain analysis, attempts have been made to create age-specific brain templates. Multicontrast, single-subject atlases for neonates and 18-month-old as well as 2-year-old children have recently been developed.[17] The low gray matter/white matter contrast in both T1- and T2-weighted MR images in young children compared with the adult brain, makes the accurate normalization of one brain to another very difficult.[17] A template-free parcellation that uses unconstrained parcellation schemes and enables calculation of single-subject network

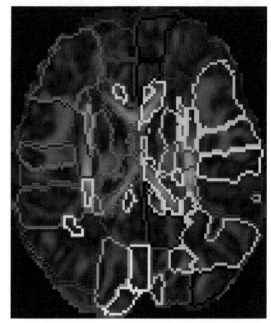

Fig. 1. Parcellations of the human brain into discrete nodes. The neonatal Johns Hopkins University (JHU) atlas is shown here.

parameters without imposing anatomic bias may be a valuable alternative and has shown promising results in the segmentation of the neonatal brain.[18]

A novel data-driven approach to explore the cortical architecture has been recently described such as Dense Individualized and Common Connectivity-based Cortical Landmarks.[19]

EDGES: BRAIN WIRING

Diffusion MR tractography is the most commonly used diffusion MR imaging method for defining structural connectivity.[16,20] At present DTI tractography is still the only in vivo tool capable of estimating structural connectivity in the brain. Fiber tractography is a rendering method for improving the depiction of 2D DTI data of the brain (Fig. 2).[21–26]

The fibers depicted with tractography are often considered to represent axonal bundles or nerve fibers, but they are more correctly viewed in physical terms as lines of fast diffusion that follow the local diffusion maxima and that only generally/mathematically reflect the axonal architecture.[27] The goal of diffusion-weighted imaging (DWI)/DTI analysis is to infer a probability function for each voxel, which captures the different fiber orientations present and their relative proportions. Estimation of this function at each voxel, which is referred to as the fiber orientation density function

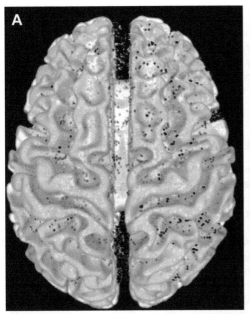
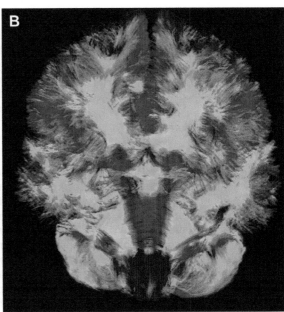

Fig. 2. Connecting the dots. (*A*) Endpoints of whole brain tractography overlaid on the brain surface. (*B*) 3D depiction of whole brain tractography obtained with HARDI of an 8-year-old healthy subject. Improved tractography with HARDI is capable of capturing more connections and yield detailed representation of the white matter, for example, edges.

(fODF), is the first step in estimating structural connectivity (Fig. 3).

The DTI model performs well in regions where there is only 1 fiber population (ie, fibers are aligned along a single axis), whereby it gives a good depiction of the fiber orientation. However, this is not always the case. Fibers are known to disperse (fan), cross, merge and kiss (temporarily run adjacent to one another), all of which can occur within the same single voxel and lead to heterogeneity not accounted for by a simple delta function. Complex fODF models better estimate fiber trajectories, particularly when several white matter tracts intersect and allow recovery of

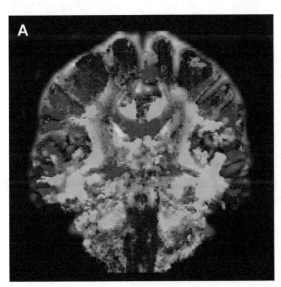
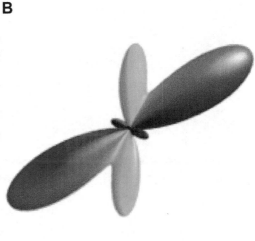

Fig. 3. (*A*) Coronal view of a directionally encoded color (DEC) map showing the major white matter fibers in 2D. (*B*) fOD. Estimations of water molecule diffusion aids in fiber tractography by recovering complex fiber-crossing configurations.

nondominant pathways invisible to DTI. Imaging techniques that provide higher angular resolution are needed.[28,29] Two newer approaches, diffusion spectrum imaging (DSI) and high-angular resolution diffusion imaging (HARDI), and their variations have begun to replace DTI in recent years. Although they differ in their details, HARDI and DSI ultimately work by detecting the movement of water in many more directions within a given voxel.[30]

After estimation of the fODF in each voxel, tractography approaches such as deterministic or probabilistic algorithms, are used to establish structural connectivity between connectome nodes.[16]

Deterministic or probabilistic tractography is applied to assign "connection" between each pair of cortical regions in the brain.[27,28,30–32]

Special considerations for children related to acquisition time and issues regarding connectivity of the developing brain have been described previously.[16]

THE CONNECTIVITY MATRIX

The next step in structural connectome reconstruction is the generation of an association matrix by compiling all pairwise associations between nodes. By applying a threshold to each element of this matrix we obtain a binary adjacency matrix or undirected graph (Fig. 4).

NETWORK METRICS

Because network analysis is based on the mathematical field of graph theory, there is a wide variety of measures that can be used to characterize the topological architecture of the brain's anatomic or functional connectivity. In particular, graphs are commonly assessed in terms of their local and global connectivity/efficiency (Table 1).[16,33] Normal brain development is characterized by continuous network changes throughout infancy, childhood, and adolescence, following specific maturational patterns. During development, the

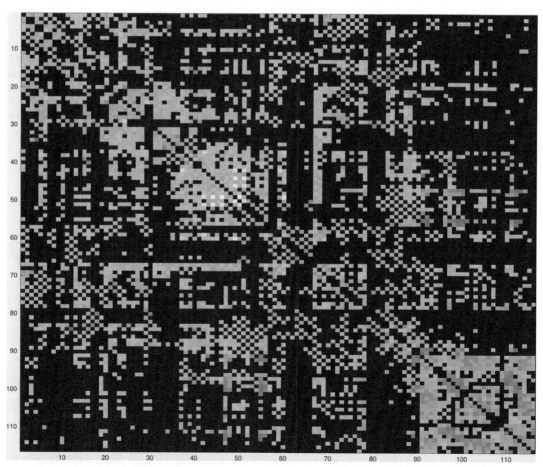

Fig. 4. Connectivity matrix. The essence of the connectome, represents the association matrix by compiling all pairwise associations (edges) between nodes.

Table 1
Network metrics

Network Metric	Definition
Measures of local connectivity	
Clustering coefficient	A measure of local segregation or efficiency, measures the density of connections between the node's neighbors
Transitivity	A normalized variant of clustering coefficient not influenced by nodes with low degree
Modularity	Decomposability of the system into smaller subsystems, eg community structure
Measures of global connectivity	
Characteristic path length	A measure of network integration, is the average shortest path length between all pairs of nodes in the network; short path is likely to be most effective for internode communication
Measures of influence and centrality	
Degree	Number of edges connecting it to the rest of the network
Hub	Important nodes highly connected to the rest of the network, facilitate global integrative processes
Between-ness centrality	Fraction of all shortest paths in the network that pass through the node
Measures of resilience	
Degree distribution	The distribution of degrees over all nodes in the network; brain graphs typically have a broad-scale degree distribution, implying that at least a few "hubs" will have high degree
Assortativity coefficient	Measure of resilience on the correlation coefficient for the degree of neighboring nodes; networks with a positive assortativity coefficient are resilient. Networks with a negative assortativity are likely vulnerable
Other	
Small-worldness	The combination of high clustering and short characteristic path length; also defined as the combination of high global and local efficiency of information transfer between nodes of a network

From Meoded A, Huisman T, Casamassima MGS, et al. The structural connectome in children: basic concepts, how to build it, and synopsis of challenges for the developing pediatric brain. Neuroradiology 2017;59:445–460.

structural connectome demonstrates increased global integration and robustness and decreased local segregation, as well as the strengthening of the hubs. Network measures can be used as diagnostic biomarkers to quantify differences between patients and healthy subjects.

ANALYSIS OF THE CONNECTOME: CONNECTOMICS

When comparing brain graphs and topology measures, it is important to observe 2 main rules: the graphs to be compared must have (1) the same number of nodes and (2) the same number of edges. This is because the quantitative values of topological metrics will depend on both the size and connection density of the graphs, and in order to identify topological differences between graphs that specifically point to the difference between groups.[4] Furthermore, building a "consensus connectome" can be created when analyzing heterogeneous groups of subjects with too much interindividual variation of structural connectivity. The consensus connectomes have the advantage of being pooled across all the individuals in the group, which smooths out individual variation

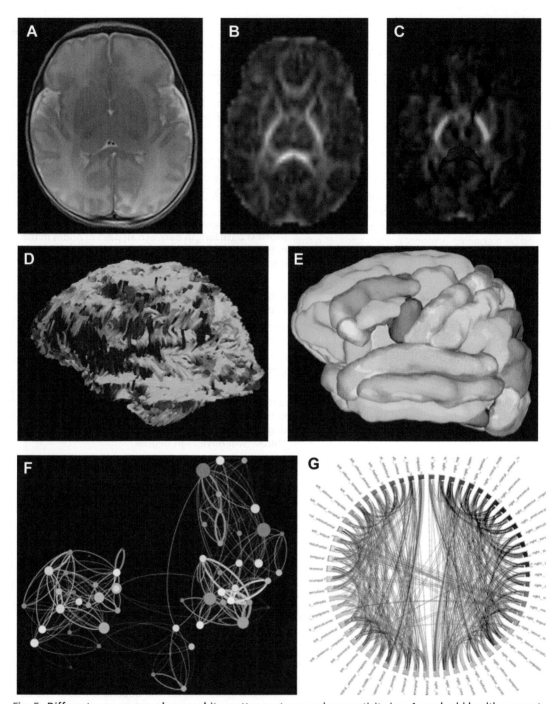

Fig. 5. Different ways we can observe white matter anatomy and connectivity in a 1-week-old healthy neonate. (*A*) Axial T2-weighted image, (*B*) axial fractional anisotropy (FA), (*C*) axial DEC map, (*D*) whole brain tractography, (*E*) cortical segmentation according to JHU atlas, (*F*) network visualization with nodes as spheres with different colors and sizes, according to modularity partitioning and hub, respectively, (*G*) circular-modules: all cortical regions depicted as rectangles with size based on degree of a module, connected by weighted edges.

and allows for comparison of graph metrics with other studies that have reported results for consensus connectomes.[14] In addition to comparing topological structures of entire graphs, one can identify subnetworks of graphs that are different between groups, for example, network-based statistics (NBS).[34] NBS has the ability to detect differences in connectivity between groups

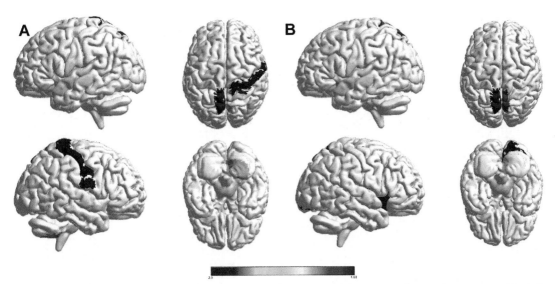

Fig. 6. Network hubs (nodes with nodal between-ness of 2 SD greater than network mean between-ness) include bilateral precuneus, right postcentral gyrus and right eighth cerebellar lobule in "virtual callosotomy" controls (A) and bilateral precuneus, bilateral insula and right lingual gyrus in patients with AgCC (B). (From Meoded A, Katipally R, Bosemani T, et al. Structural connectivity analysis reveals abnormal brain connections in agenesis of the corpus callosum in children. Eur Radiol 2015;25:1471–8; with permission.)

and may be helpful in identifying alternate wiring or reorganization of brain networks.[13]

NETWORK VISUALIZATION

The increase interest and popularity in the human connectome, has established a new neuroimaging dimension: the imaging of networks (Fig. 5). The dimensionality of human connectivity data is high and the complex networks require sophisticated visualization and analysis software.[35] Innovations in data visualization exemplify the landmark advances in human connectome research since its origins including glyphs for DWI/DTI and graph-based brain network representations of structural connectivity data.[36] The result in any connectome visualization is a trade-off between anatomic fidelity and connectome complexity. These challenges require a balance between complexity and simplicity and between thoroughness and readability.[36]

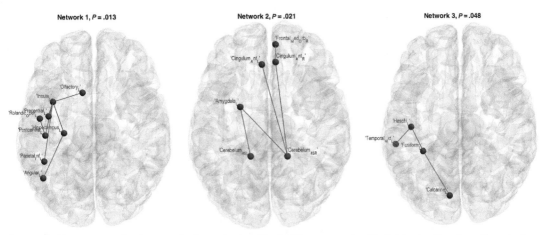

Fig. 7. Highly connected subnetworks in patients with AgCC compared with "virtual callosotomy" controls as identified by network-based statistics. Networks 1 and 3 are left intrahemispheric and network 2 is interhemispheric and connects the left cerebral hemisphere with the contralateral cerebellum. (From Meoded A, Katipally R, Bosemani T, et al. Structural connectivity analysis reveals abnormal brain connections in agenesis of the corpus callosum in children. Eur Radiol 2015;25:1471–8; with permission.)

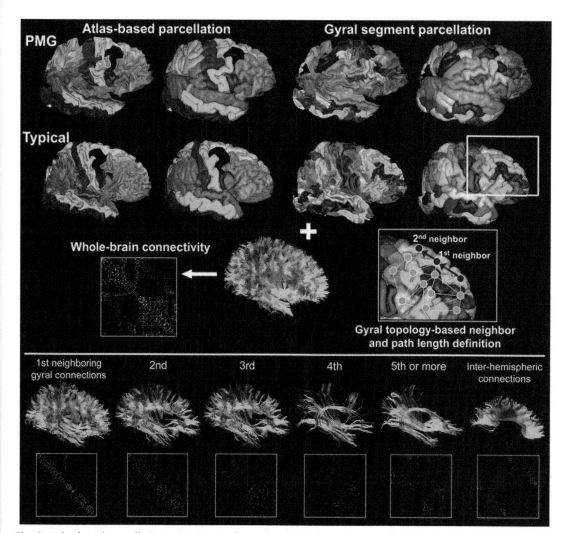

Fig. 8. Atlas-based parcellation using FreeSurfer and individual gyral pattern-based parcellation for the typical control and patients with PMG brains, and network construction for different fiber groups divided by gyral topology-based path length. The PMG shows irregular gyral patterns with abnormally oriented gyri. Anatomic parcellation and labeling using an atlas seems not proper for the PMG brain. The gyral-based segmentation provides a more uniform and consistent segmentation of both normal and PMG brains with regions that are similar in size and with equal respect for gyral topology. (*From* Im K, Paldino MJ, Poduri A, et al. Altered white matter connectivity and network organization in polymicrogyria revealed by individual gyral topology-based analysis. NeuroImage 2014;86:182–93; with permission.)

THE POTENTIAL USE OF CONNECTOMICS TO STUDY CONGENITAL BRAIN MALFORMATIONS

The structural connectome is an ideal tool to study connectivity of the malformed brain. Beyond the evident morphologic anomaly seen in conventional/anatomic MR imaging, connectomics can show the altered wiring diagram or neuroplasticity/reorganization patterns at a network level.

Connectomics has great potential for elucidating abnormal connectivity in congenital brain malformations and may provide us with a unique opportunity to study the functional response of the brain to an underlying developmental abnormality.

The structural connectome has been applied to study brain malformations, especially axonal pathfinding disorders, such as commissural anomalies.[13,37,38] Connectopathies are now considered separate, well-defined group of disorders.

Neurodevelopmental disorders are currently considered connectopathies, disorders where multiple circuits/networks throughout the cortex are involved. Thus, connectomics has the potential to enhance our understanding of and potentially aid in the diagnosis and treatment of these disorders.

Agenesis of the corpus callosum (AgCC) is one of the most common human brain malformations. AgCC can be considered a prototype of axon guidance disorder.[14]

Using graph theory approach with virtual callosotomy as a control group, Meoded and colleagues[13] showed abnormal brain connections in AgCC in children. They found reduced global and increased local connectivity in children with AgCC compared with controls. The bilateral insula were identified as hubs in patients, whereas the cerebellum was detected as a hub only in controls. In addition, 3 subnetworks of increased connectivity were identified in patients. This study suggested that neural plasticity in AgCC may attempt to increase the interhemispheric connectivity through alternative decussating pathways other than the corpus callosum (Figs. 6 and 7).

A study by Severino and colleagues[37] illustrated 3 malformative subtypes of segmental callosal agenesis. They showed that even the absence of a small callosal segment may impact global brain connectivity and modularity organization.

Finally, using individual gyral topology-based analysis Im and colleagues[39] reported altered white matter connectivity and network organization in patients with polymicrogyria (PMG). In this study, the author examined structural connectivity and network topology of 14 PMG subjects using individual primary gyral pattern-based nodes in patients with PMG, overcoming the limitations of an atlas-based approach (Fig. 8). This study showed the potential for an individualized method to characterize network properties and alterations in connections that are associated with malformations of cortical development.

CONCLUSION AND FUTURE DIRECTIONS

In this review article, we outlined the different steps and the many challenges that remain in the acquisition, processing and analysis of the structural connectome in children. The measurement of the network topology allows a better understanding of the pathogenesis, implication for cognitive and behavioral functions, and treatment of pediatric brain disorders from a network perspective. Innovative methods of neuroimaging data analysis are essential for the structural connectome. Brain connectomics is becoming a core component of several neuroscience research projects. In summary, the human connectome provides an unparalleled compilation of neural

data allowing to navigate the brain and explore developing brain circuits in a way that was not possible in the preconnectome era. Neurodevelopmental disorders, including congenital brain malformations can be better explored with a network-based approach.

REFERENCES

1. Craddock RC, Jbabdi S, Yan CG, et al. Imaging human connectomes at the macroscale. Nat Methods 2013;10:524–39.
2. Sporns O, Tononi G, Kotter R. The human connectome: a structural description of the human brain. PLoS Comput Biol 2005;1:e42.
3. Bullmore E, Sporns O. Complex brain networks: graph theoretical analysis of structural and functional systems. Nat Rev Neurosci 2009;10:186–98.
4. Bullmore ET, Bassett DS. Brain graphs: graphical models of the human brain connectome. Annu Rev Clin Psychol 2011;7:113–40.
5. Erdos P, Renyi A. On the evolution of random graphs. B Int Statist Inst 1960;38:343–7.
6. Papo D, Buldu JM, Boccaletti S, et al. Complex network theory and the brain. Philos Trans R Soc Lond B Biol Sci 2014;369. https://doi.org/10.1098/rstb.2013.0520.
7. Sporns O. The human connectome: a complex network. Ann N Y Acad Sci 2011;1224:109–25.
8. Albert R, Barabasi AL. Statistical mechanics of complex networks. Rev Mod Phys 2002;74:47–97.
9. Bassett DS, Bullmore ET. Human brain networks in health and disease. Curr Opin Neurol 2009;22:340–7.
10. Latora V, Marchiori M. Efficient behavior of small-world networks. Phys Rev Lett 2001;87:198701.
11. Watts DJ, Strogatz SH. Collective dynamics of 'small-world' networks. Nature 1998;393:440–2.
12. Sporns O, Zwi JD. The small world of the cerebral cortex. Neuroinformatics 2004;2:145–62.
13. Meoded A, Katipally R, Bosemani T, et al. Structural connectivity analysis reveals abnormal brain connections in agenesis of the corpus callosum in children. Eur Radiol 2015;25:1471–8.
14. Owen JP, Li YO, Ziv E, et al. The structural connectome of the human brain in agenesis of the corpus callosum. Neurolmage 2013;70:340–55.
15. Widjaja E, Zamyadi M, Raybaud C, et al. Disrupted global and regional structural networks and subnetworks in children with localization-related epilepsy. AJNR Am J Neuroradiol 2015;36:1362–8.
16. Meoded A, Huisman T, Casamassima MGS, et al. The structural connectome in children: basic concepts, how to build it, and synopsis of challenges for the developing pediatric brain. Neuroradiology 2017;59:445–60.
17. Oishi K, Mori S, Donohue PK, et al. Multi-contrast human neonatal brain atlas: application to normal

neonate development analysis. NeuroImage 2011; 56:8–20.

18. Tymofiyeva O, Hess CP, Ziv E, et al. Towards the "baby connectome": mapping the structural connectivity of the newborn brain. PLoS One 2012;7: e31029.

19. Zhu D, Li K, Terry DP, et al. Connectome-scale assessments of structural and functional connectivity in MCI. Hum Brain Mapp 2014;35:2911–23.

20. Mori S, Zhang J. Principles of diffusion tensor imaging and its applications to basic neuroscience research. Neuron 2006;51:527–39.

21. Le Bihan D. Molecular diffusion, tissue microdynamics and microstructure. NMR Biomed 1995;8: 375–86.

22. Mori S, Crain BJ, Chacko VP, et al. Three-dimensional tracking of axonal projections in the brain by magnetic resonance imaging. Ann Neurol 1999;45: 265–9.

23. Basser PJ, Mattiello J, LeBihan D. MR diffusion tensor spectroscopy and imaging. Biophys J 1994; 66:259–67.

24. Conturo TE, Lori NF, Cull TS, et al. Tracking neuronal fiber pathways in the living human brain. Proc Natl Acad Sci U S A 1999;96:10422–7.

25. Pierpaoli C, Jezzard P, Basser PJ, et al. Diffusion tensor MR imaging of the human brain. Radiology 1996;201:637–48.

26. Pierpaoli C, Basser PJ. Toward a quantitative assessment of diffusion anisotropy. Magn Reson Med 1996;36:893–906.

27. Hagmann P, Jonasson L, Maeder P, et al. Understanding diffusion MR imaging techniques: from scalar diffusion-weighted imaging to diffusion tensor imaging and beyond. Radiographics 2006;26(Suppl 1):S205–23.

28. Tuch DS, Reese TG, Wiegell MR, et al. High angular resolution diffusion imaging reveals intravoxel white matter fiber heterogeneity. Magn Reson Med 2002; 48:577–82.

29. Basser PJ, Mattiello J, LeBihan D. Estimation of the effective self-diffusion tensor from the NMR spin echo. J Magn Reson B 1994;103:247–54.

30. Wedeen VJ, Hagmann P, Tseng WY, et al. Mapping complex tissue architecture with diffusion spectrum magnetic resonance imaging. Magn Reson Med 2005;54:1377–86.

31. Hagmann P, Grant PE, Fair DA. MR connectomics: a conceptual framework for studying the developing brain. Front Syst Neurosci 2012;6:43.

32. Tournier JD, Calamante F, Connelly A. Robust determination of the fibre orientation distribution in diffusion MRI: non-negativity constrained super-resolved spherical deconvolution. NeuroImage 2007;35:1459–72.

33. Rubinov M, Sporns O. Complex network measures of brain connectivity: uses and interpretations. NeuroImage 2010;52:1059–69.

34. Zalesky A, Fornito A, Bullmore ET. Network-based statistic: identifying differences in brain networks. NeuroImage 2010;53:1197–207.

35. LaPlante RA, Douw L, Tang W, et al. The connectome visualization utility: software for visualization of human brain networks. PLoS One 2014;9: e113838.

36. Margulies DS, Bottger J, Watanabe A, et al. Visualizing the human connectome. NeuroImage 2013; 80:445–61.

37. Severino M, Tortora D, Toselli B, et al. Structural connectivity analysis in children with segmental callosal agenesis. AJNR Am J Neuroradiol 2017;38(3): 639–47.

38. Barch DM, Burgess GC, Harms MP, et al. Function in the human connectome: task-fMRI and individual differences in behavior. NeuroImage 2013;80: 169–89.

39. Im K, Paldino MJ, Poduri A, et al. Altered white matter connectivity and network organization in polymicrogyria revealed by individual gyral topology-based analysis. NeuroImage 2014;86:182–93.

Corpus Callosum
Molecular Pathways in Mice and Human Dysgeneses

Charles Raybaud, MD, FRCPC

KEYWORDS

- Corpus callosum • Development • Midline guidance molecules • Midline zipper • Indusium griseum
- Glial wedge

KEY POINTS

- Commissures connect homologous structures of either sides along the central nervous system.
- It is generally assumed that cross-wiring results from the physics of vision: the retinal image being inverted by the lens, the chiasmatic decussation restores the continuity of the image in the topographically organized cortex.
- Although some connections of the corpus callosum are known to be heterotopic, a large heterotopic callosal bundle (the so-called sigmoid bundle) is not classically described in normal anatomic studies.

Commissures connect homologous structures of either sides along the central nervous system (CNS). Although it is not proven, it is generally assumed that cross-wiring results from the physics of vision: the retinal image being inverted by the lens, the chiasmatic decussation restores the continuity of the image in the topographically organized cortex; tactile crossing then is needed to allow easy integration of the sensory inputs, and motor crossing, to allow prompt motor response (Ramon y Cajal, quoted by[1]). As a step further, commissures are needed for bilateral integration and better body coordination. Whereas the evolutionarily oldest anterior and hippocampal commissures are found in all mammals, a corpus callosum is found in placental mammals only.[2–4] Both the anterior (paleocortical) and the hippocampal commissures cross the midline in a very simple way at the level of the lamina reuniens of His (upper portion of the lamina terminalis), where the 2 hemispheres are in continuity.[5] They include, respectively, fibers of the anterior–inferior temporal, and posterior parietooccipitotemporal neocortex. On the contrary, the frontal neocortical fibers (anterior corpus callosum) need an interhemispheric glial and neuronal bridging structure to guide and support the crossing fibers along the cortical boundary of the septum pellucidum.[6,7]

ANATOMY OF THE TELENCEPHALIC COMMISSURES

In the modern understanding of the organization of the CNS the telencephalon is the dorsal part of the secondary prosencephalon. It derives from the anterior neural plate (ANP), the part of the neuroectoderm that extends rostral to the notochord and includes the future hemispheres and basal ganglia (classic telencephalon) as well as the anterior, hypothalamic part of the third ventricle.[8] The hemispheres become connected by a commissural arch made of the 3 main telencephalic commissures: the anterior commissure, the hippocampal commissure and the corpus callosum, which itself includes an anterior callosum, which surrounds the septum pellucidum, and a splenium that overlies the hippocampal commissure.

The author has nothing to disclose.
99 Harbour Square #1102, Toronto, Ontario M5J2H2, Canada
E-mail address: charles.raybaud@gmail.com

Neuroimag Clin N Am 29 (2019) 445–459
https://doi.org/10.1016/j.nic.2019.03.006

The anterior commissure crosses the midline at the upper end of the lamina terminalis, anterior to the foramen of Monro, within the bifurcation of the fornix into its precommissural (septal) and postcommissural (mammillary) tracts. It extends laterally in the depth of the anterior portion of the basal ganglia, connecting the amygdalae and the septal nuclei. It contains approximately 3.5 million fibers in humans; its diameter is never greater than 6 mm (author's personal data). It is made of 2 components separated by a well-defined glial plane.[9] The anterior component is paleocortical and consists of small unmyelinated fibers mostly; it connects the olfactory structures (olfactory bulbs, septal nuclei, and amygdalae). The posterior component, made of small myelinated fibers, connects some orbitofrontal and insular neocortex,[10] as well as most of the associative anterior, lateral, and inferior temporal neocortex.[9,11]

Thought for long to be only residual in humans, the hippocampal commissure is now proven to be functional, based on electrophysiologic, clinical, and anatomic data.[12–17] It connects the mesial temporal cortices across the midline. Most mammals present 2 hippocampal commissures: one ventral that corresponds with the body of the fornix, and one dorsal, with the crura. Gloor and colleagues[17] demonstrated that in humans and other primates the ventral hippocampal commissure is at most vestigial, and that the dorsal hippocampal commissure connects the bilateral presubiculum, entorhinal, and parahippocampal cortices, but not the hippocampus proper: it is, therefore, a truly parahippocampal, purely neocortical commissure. It is a part of the fornix: the mesial temporal fibers gather in the fimbriae, and form the crura of the fornices around the choroid fissures and thalami, before joining each other on the midline in the lower edge of the septal leaves to form the body of the fornix; at the level of the anterior commissure, each column of the fornix divides into a precommissural, hippocamposeptal tract that connects to the septal nuclei, and a postcommissural tract that contains subicular fibers and connects to the mammillary bodies. Although 80% of the fibers remain ipsilateral, about 20% cross the midline and form the (dorsal) hippocampal commissure between the forniceal crura, a transverse triangular structure with an anterior apex that abuts the posterior end of the forniceal body (ie, of the septum pellucidum), a posterior base transversely attached to the ventral aspect of the callosal splenium/forceps major, and a midline attachment to the undersurface of the callosal splenium. In monkeys, the hippocampal commissure consists of small myelinated neocortical fibers; it is clearly separated from the callosal

splenium by a glial plane.[9] Also, a small number of hippocampal fibers decussate along the forniceal bodies to join the contralateral septal area (hippocampal decussation) in addition to the hippocampal commissure.[15]

The corpus callosum is the most prominent forebrain commissure in advanced mammals, spanning much of the frontal and parietal lobes from the anterior commissure ventrally to behind the hippocampal commissure dorsally. It is made of 200 to 300 million fibers, mostly thick, well-myelinated axons posteriorly (connecting the primary cortices), and mostly thin, thinly myelinated fibers anteriorly (connecting the associative frontal cortices). In a similar way, functionally as well as developmentally, it can be divided into an anterior, frontal callosum and a callosal splenium separated by a focal narrowing or isthmus, which corresponds with the central sulcus and sensory motor cortex (as demonstrated by modern diffusion tensor imaging tractography studies).[18] The anterior callosum, therefore, corresponds with the frontal and anterior cingulate cortices, whereas the splenium corresponds with the parietal, occipital, and posterior temporal cortices, and the posterior cingulate gyrus. The anterior callosum is associated with, and surrounds, the septum pellucidum, whereas the splenium overlies the hippocampal commissure. It does not exist in monotremes and marsupials, in which all neocortical commissural axons instead cross together with the fibers of the anterior and hippocampal commissures.

The anterior callosum can be further divided into segments that reflect the cortical organization of the frontal lobe: clockwise, from the anterior commissure, those segments are (1) the semihorizontal lamina rostralis/rostrum that extends anteriorly from the anterior commissure to the inferior–posterior aspect of the genu and separates the septal area ventrally (subcallosal gyrus) from the septum pellucidum dorsally, already visible in the fetus at 14 weeks,[19] it is likely to connect the frontobasal cortices on either side[18,20]; (2) the thick genu (knee) marks the abrupt change in orientation between the lamina rostralis and the callosal body and corresponds to the anterior apex of the septum pellucidum—it contains the forceps minor that connects the bilateral prefrontal cortices and anterior cingulate gyri[18]; (3) the horizontal callosal body extends from the callosal genu to the isthmus—it borders the septum pellucidum superiorly while laterally its fibers form the roofs of the lateral ventricular bodies and connect the precentral/premotor cortices, the adjacent insular gyri, and the corresponding cingulate gyri[18,20]; and (4) last, the isthmus is a focal narrowing that contains the commissural fibers of the precentral and postcentral gyri[18,20] and of the primary auditory area[3,21,22]—this is where the fornix joins the undersurface of the corpus callosum.

The splenium (spleen), the thickest portion of the corpus callosum, protrudes in the ambient cistern and overhangs the tectal plate; the vein of Galen sweeps around it. Its morphology is extremely variable, from rounded to flat. It should be located above or just at the line drawn along the third ventricular floor; not uncommonly, it drops below this line in cases of idiopathic developmental delay.[22] The splenial fibers form the forceps major and participate in the tapetum, or sagittal stratum, in the lateral wall of the ventricular atrium. They can be subdivided into a superior group that contains the fibers of the posterior parietal cortex, a posterior group that contains the fibers of the medial occipital cortex, and an inferior group that contains the fibers of the posterior temporal cortex.[3,18,20] Along the midline, the hippocampal commissure is attached to the undersurface of the splenium.

The septum pellucidum is roughly triangular, located above the lamina rostralis, surrounded by the anterior callosum anterosuperiorly, with the body of the fornix running in its lower edge. It closes the medial aspect of the body of the lateral ventricles. Abbie[2] and Rakic and Yakovlev[6] strongly emphasized that the nature of the septum pellucidum is closely related to the development of the corpus callosum. Its detailed anatomy is not well-known. From a terminologic point of view it is often confused with the paleopallial septum granulosum (part of the olfactory cortex), a gray matter structure that is located inferior to the lamina rostralis and anterior to the lamina terminalis and the hypothalamus; it is made of 2 nuclei associated with the diagonal band of Broca, one medial (the subcallosal gyrus) and one deeper in the hemisphere. By contrast, the septum pellucidum is made of 2 sheaths of white matter, ependyma lined on their ventricular surface, but with no organized gray matter[23–25]; it has been shown to carry axonal fibers in rats,[26] monkeys,[27] and humans[28] which form the fanning septocingulate perforating pathway[26] that connects the medial septum and diagonal band of Broca to the cingulate cortex, intersecting (hence the epithet "perforating") the corpus callosum along the way; it also contains a bundle of cingulothalamic perforant fibers.[27] Within its lower edge, the septum pellucidum contains the joined columns of the fornix that, connecting the septal nuclei with the mesial temporal structures, may be considered anatomically the mesiotemporal equivalent of the frontoparietal septocingulate perforating pathway.

DEVELOPMENT OF THE TELENCEPHALIC COMMISSURES

As mentioned, the telencephalic hemispheres are part of the secondary prosencephalon,[8] which includes the hypothalamic part of the third ventricle, the basal ganglia (subpallium), and the pallium itself (cortex and associated white matter). The pallium in turn comprises the paleocortex (septal nuclei and amygdala), the archicortex (hippocampal formation), and the neocortex; the development of the telencephalic commissures reflects this organization. The secondary prosencephalon derives from the rostral-most portion of the neuroectoderm that develops anterior to the notochord, above the pharyngeal membrane, and forms, at the beginning of the fourth week, the ANP. The circumference of the ANP is called the anterior neural ridge (ANR). The ANR expresses Fgf8 and is considered the organizer of the telencephalon, just like the midbrain–hindbrain isthmus is the organizer of the brainstem.[29] During the fourth week, the ANP becomes surrounded by neural crest cells (mesectoderm) while it closes to form the secondary prosencephalon. The closure line corresponds with the apposition of the lips of the ANR on the dorsal midline. Still expressing Fgf8, these lips become the bilateral hem on either side of the midline, still a telencephalic organizer (together with a pallial–subpallial antihem laterally). The hem medially induces the development of the tela choroidea and, laterally, the development of a hippocampal primordium (and eventually a large part of the cortex), by giving rise to the earliest neurons of the cortex, the Cajal-Retzius cells.[30] From week 6 onward, the lesser growth of the medial tela choroidea as compared with the lateral hemispheric vesicles results in the so-called interhemispheric invagination, that is, the future interhemispheric fissure.

The hem itself is not cortical, in the way that it will not become integrated in the medial cortex.[30] Being interposed between the tela choroidea and the pallium, it corresponds with a parasagittal medullary velum in which the early fimbria and fornix develop (weeks 8–10) and forms the primitive, still Fgf8-expressing septum pellucidum.[31,32] It is continuous anteriorly with the thickened upper portion of the lamina terminalis that forms the lamina reuniens (linking plate), the direct connection between the hemispheres where the paleocortical and archicortical commissural fibers cross to form the corresponding basal telencephalic (future anterior) and hippocampal commissures (weeks 8–11 in humans). In monotremes and marsupials, all neocortical fibers eventually travel alongside these 2 commissures. In eutherians (placental), only temporal, occipital, and parietal neocortical commissural fibers follow the basal telencephalic and hippocampal commissures as well, to complete the anterior commissure and form the splenium (weeks 8–13). All frontal commissural fibers instead cross using a line of secondary fusion of the medial hemispheric walls. This fusion occurs at the boundary between the septum pellucidum and the cortex (corticoseptal boundary)[6,7] (Fig. 1A), and results from the migration of glial cells (zipper glia) and neurons (neuronal sling). There the frontal commissural fibers cross the midline, first from the cingulate, then from the more lateral cortices, isolating ventrally the bilaminar septum pellucidum from the more dorsal, cortex-lined interhemispheric fissure in the process. These fibers are conveyed toward the midline by the repulsive action of a dorsal, interhemispheric *indusium griseum* glia and a ventral, ventricular glial wedge. When approaching the inner aspect of the hemisphere the fibers become attracted by the bridging midline glial zipper and a 3-layered neuronal sling (see Fig. 1B). All together, these structures form the cellular midline guideposts that allow pioneer cingulate (paralimbic) commissural fibers to cross. Both glial and neuronal components derive from the mesial ventricular/subventricular zones by early specification of neuroglial progenitors. Because this occurs along the corticoseptal boundary, the anterior (frontal) callosum is anatomically associated with the septum pellucidum (weeks 11–13). At the same time, other fibers originating from the septum granulosum (septal cortex) extend cranially within the ipsilateral leaf of the septum pellucidum to connect with the ipsilateral cingulate cortex, perpendicularly to the crossing callosal fiber, making up the septocingulate perforating bundle, which composes the mature septum

pellucidum together with the fornix in its lower edge. With the continuing development of the lateral neocortical frontal cortex, additional callosal fibers from the more lateral frontal neocortex can cross by fasciculating along the initial cingulate pioneer fibers to complete the anterior callosum, from the temporal neocortex along the basal telencephalic commissure to form the final anterior commissure, and from the posterior parietooccipital neocortex along the hippocampal commissure to form the callosal splenium. At the same time, the midline guidepost apparatus regresses and disappears, leaving a cavitation between the leaves of the septum pellucidum and below the anterior callosum, the cavum septi pellucidi.[33] This cavum typically closes progressively by a back-to-front apposition of its leaves until about the time of birth (for details regarding the morphogenesis of the commissures see[34]).

MOLECULAR SIGNALING OF COMMISSURAL MORPHOGENESIS

Commissures and decussations cross the midline everywhere along the CNS, which involves complex processes of neuronal specification, axonal selection and guidance, midline crossing signaling and bundle formation (see[5] for a review). Because of the functional importance of the telencephalon, and the clinical significance of the syndromes of callosal agenesis, special attention was paid to the telencephalic commissures in the last few decades. This review tries to summarize the molecular processes that have been shown to be associated with the development of the dorsal telencephalic commissures. Several steps should be considered. (1) The interhemispheric midline should be well-formed and permissive. (2) Specific populations of commissural neurons should be

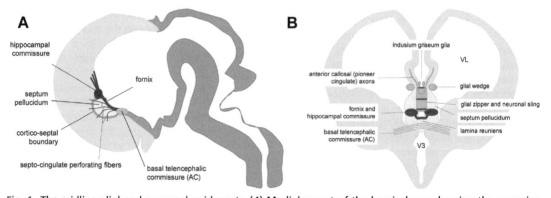

Fig. 1. The midline glial and neuronal guideposts. (*A*) Medial aspect of the hemispheres showing the organization of the midline white matter tracts in relation to the septum pellucidum. (*B*) Coronal cut of the telencephalon showing the organization of the midline guideposts and crossing commissures. AC, anterior commissure; VL, ventrolateral.

able to differentiate from the progenitor population, to migrate properly to specific locations, and to develop a commissural branch rather than, or in addition to, a projection branch; in addition, proper guidance molecules and their receptors should direct this commissural branch toward the midline. (3) The interhemispheric fissure must have remodeled in a way to provide a bridge for the crossing commissural axons: migration of midline glial and neuronal guideposts and production of appropriate guidance factors. (4) Post-crossing pioneer axons must be able to find their way toward their final destination beyond the attractive midline. Finally (5), later neocortical commissural axons should be able to fasciculate along the pioneer cingulate axons. Importantly, most data have been collected in mice; they explain the morphogenesis well, but nevertheless they may not be directly applicable for understanding the human malformations.

Development of the Interhemispheric Fissure

The dorsal telencephalic commissures develop in combination with the process of division of the telencephalon in 2 hemispheres. The telencephalon originate from the ANP. The ANP extends rostrally beyond the notochord and the cranial extension of the mesoderm, so that the cranial perineural mesenchyme (or mesectoderm) originates from the cranial neural crest (CNC) that migrates from the mesodiencephalic neural crest and not from the somitic mesoderm. The CNC ultimately forms the supratentorial meninges, membranous skull and scalp, as well as the face and anterior skull base. In addition, it plays a major role in the development, closure, and organization of the ANP.[29] Its surrounding ANR is considered the telencephalic organizer and expresses *Fgf8*; this expression depends on the presence of the CNC and, in turn, *Fgf8* attracts the migrating cells of the CNC. The activation of *Fgf8* results in the upregulation of *Gremlin* and *Noggin*, which are antagonists of the *BMP* signaling molecules (notably *Bmp4*) expressed in the neighboring ectoderm, which would repress the expression of *Fgf8*.[29,35] The presence of CNC cells seems to be critical for the closure of the anterior forebrain as well, through a mechanism not elucidated yet, as well as for the dorsalization of the prosencephalic alar plate by upregulating the dorsalization factor *Wnt8b*.[35] Through the process of closure of the forebrain vesicle, the lateral ANR join each other along the dorsal midline to form a bilateral hem, and the rostromedial fold forms the lamina reuniens. The hem retains the organizing expression of *Fgf8*, which persists in its final derivative the septum pellucidum.[31,32] The hem is a major source of *Wnt1;Wnt3a* that activates the expansion of the neural crest derivatives such as the meninges. It activates the telencephalic division by inducing medially the differentiation of the tela choroidea and laterally, the production of the Cajal-Retzius cells, which initiate the formation of the cerebral cortex.[36] Between the tela choroidea and the cortex, the hem forms a medullary velum that becomes the septum pellucidum, where the fornix, septocingulate perforating bundle, and corpus callosum develop. By secreting *BMP7*, the leptomeninges initially prevent the callosal axons to grow into the interhemispheric fissure; however, this inhibition will be overcome when *Wnt3* becomes expressed in the commissural neurons of the cingulate cortex. Wnt3 expression in turn is regulated by *GDF5*, another BNP family member produced by the adjacent Cajal-Retzius cells, itself regulated by the inhibitor *Dan* produced by the meninges.[37] Also, *Netrin1 (Ntn1)* seems to be promoting the interhemispheric meningeal removal needed for the development of the glial and neuronal guideposts by promoting the disruption of the meningeal laminin: in mice lacking *Ntn1*, the callosal axons fail to extend to the midline.[38]

Layer and Axonal Specification of Callosal Neurons

Anatomically in mice, about 20% of callosal projection neurons (CPNs) are found in layer 5, and 80% in layers 2 to 3.[39] All of course extend commissural axons, but they are different neurons with different connections. In mice, and presumably also in humans, the deep layer CPNs, presumably evolutionarily older, tend to present a dual axonal branching with an ipsilateral branch projecting to the internal capsule in addition to the commissural branch. These deep layer CPNs typically establish long distance connections, to the striatum or the frontal or sensory motor cortices, ipsilaterally or contralaterally, both homotopic and heterotopic.[39] By contrast the superficial layer CPNs, evolutionarily more recent, are more exclusively commissural, with rich local collaterals to the superficial layers and still more, to the deep layers 5 and 6, as well as homotopic collaterals into the contralateral cortex.[39] These anatomic differences of the CPNs necessarily reflect different molecular signaling pathways, regarding their cortical distribution, their local or long-distance connections ipsilaterally, and their homotopic and heterotopic connections contralaterally. Nevertheless, most experimental data apply to the CPNs of the superficial layers only.

An important step in the study of the population of CPNs was the identification of a commissural neuronal maker: all commissural neurons express *Satb2*, a DNA binding protein that regulates the organization of the chromatin (and therefore the gene expression) of CPNs by repressing *CTIP2*, another transcription factor that is known to be critical for the development and fasciculation of the projection axon of the corticospinal motor neurons.[39,40] The somatosensory callosal neurons of layers 2 to 3 are specified early in the subventricular zone by the expression of *Cited2*, yet, CPNs and the corresponding glia seem to result from a delayed generation of a specific fate-restricted populations of radial glial progenitors.[41] The transcription factor *Neurogenin2* (*Ngn2*) promotes the pyramidal fate of the callosal neuron (glutamate expression, radial migration to the cortical layers 2 and 3, and axonal/dendritic morphology) as well as the decision for the axon to project medially toward the commissural plate rather than laterally toward subcortical or ipsilateral cortical targets. It seems that this decision is made very early during neuronal differentiation, well before the neurons reach their final location in layers 2 and 3.[42] Obviously, the genetic control of the neuronal migration and cortical organization is important, because genetic mutations that result in an abnormal migration may also result in callosal agenesis/dysgenesis. This applies to the neuronal cytoskeleton, because it is central to the processes of cell proliferation, migration, and connection; callosal dysgenesis is highly prevalent in tubulinopathies.[43,44] The migration of the CPNs and their positioning in the superficial layers have been shown to depend on *FILIP* (Filamin interacting protein).[45] Dendritic differentiation is compromised in neurons with mutated *COUP-TFI* gene because of a decreased expression of its downstream effector *MAP1B* (microtubule-associated protein); commissural axons of the hippocampal and callosal commissures fail to cross while the anterior commissure demonstrates abnormal connections.[46]

Building up an interhemispheric midline bridge The evolutionarily older anterior and hippocampal commissures cross in the anterior lamina reuniens. In contrast, the pioneer cingulate commissural axons need the 2 hemispheres to become fused along the junction line between the cortex and the septum pellucidum (the corticoseptal boundary). Interhemispheric fusion first implies the removal of the meninges and, then, the development of a complex midline astroglial and neuronal structure. The bridging midline glia (interhemispheric) is designated the midline zipper glia. Its dorsal surface is covered with what used to be called the glial sling, actually a mostly neuronal structure,[47] and is part of what is now identified as the neuronal guidepost. In mice, the midline zipper astroglia differentiate from the subventricular radial glia in the early fetal period,[5] and in humans at about week 8, long before the rest of the hemispheric glia (end of second trimester in man). Commissural axonal fibers are funneled toward this bridge by the indusium griseum glia, located just above the future callosum on the medial aspect of the mantle, and by the glial wedge, a periventricular structure made of radial glia that have lost their connection to the pia, and located below the future corpus callosum on the medial aspect of the ventricular wall.[48] Both indusium griseum glia and glial wedge express *Slit2*, a secreted extracellular matrix protein that acts as an axonal repellent. In addition to these midline glia populations, glutamatergic neurons (from the ventricular zone) and gamma-aminobutyric acid (GABA)-ergic neurons (from the medial and caudal ganglionic eminence) migrate into the glial sling and mix with the zipper glia to participate in the guidance processes.[49] In mice, the resulting commissural plate is induced by *Fgf8*, and includes 4 fields corresponding with the traversing bundles, each with a specific combination of molecular expressions: subpallial marker *SIX3* for the anterior commissural field, subpallial markers *SIX3* and *ZIC2* plus *NFIA* for the forniceal field, pallial markers *NFIA* and *EMX1* plus *ZIC2* for the hippocampal commissural field, and pallial markers *NFIA* and *EMX1* for the callosal field.[31]

Molecular control of the midline glia Fibroblast growth factor receptor 1 (FGFR1) is a major contributor in the development of the midline glia. In mice lacking FGFR1, the radial glia maintain an attachment to the ventricular wall and fail to translocate properly to the pia to form the midline astroglial zipper; the indusium griseum and the glial wedge are disrupted as well.[50] As a consequence, the callosal axons fail to cross the midline and instead are rerouted parasagittally into the septum pellucidum to form Probst's bundles. All 4 *NFI* (Nuclear Factor I) genes are expressed in the developing forebrain in mice. In the absence of *Nfia*, callosal agenesis, hydrocephalus and decreased glial fibrillary associated protein expression (a glial marker) are observed; the midline zipper astroglial cells are produced, but fail to form a midline bridge, migrating instead into the septum, while the glial population of the indusium griseum and glial wedge is reduced.[51] *Nfib* is needed as well; in mice lacking this factor, the differentiation of the radial glia into astrocytes fails to occur.[52] The expression of Nfi that results in the differentiation of the astroglia depends on the septal Fgfr8 expression, and the astroglia remodels the interhemispheric fissure by degrading the leptomeninges. Bone morphogenetic protein 7 (Bmp7), a member of the transforming growth factor-β superfamily of secreted proteins, is expressed in the region occupied by the glial wedge, the indusium griseum, and the subcallosal sling and is required for their correct development; its genetic inactivation in mice results in a marked reduction and disorganization of the 3 structures.[53] Gli3 (glioma-associated oncogene family zinc finger 3) is a transcription factor that is needed in the pallial Emx1-expressing progenitors for an appropriate telencephalic patterning; consequently, it is needed for the proper positioning of the midline glia, especially the glial wedge. In Gli3-deficient mice, the glial wedge cells translocate to the pia instead of sitting in the ventricular wall so that the callosal axons cannot cross[54]; this involves an upregulation of Slit2 expression and an altered Fgf and canonical Wnt signaling.[55] Finally, in addition to its usual role as an axonal repellent in association with the Robo receptors, the extracellular matrix protein Slit is also important for the development of the midline glial guideposts themselves; mutations of Slit1 and Slit2 in the mouse result in the indusium griseum being dislocated ventral to the glial wedge with consequent failure of the corpus callosum to develop normally.[56] Similarly, other than acting as a repellent, Draxin is needed for the indusium griseum glia to develop properly.[5]

Molecular control of the neuronal guideposts The presence of neuronal cells associated with the midline glia was first observed in 2003.[47] They include a population of immature (calretinin positive) glutamatergic cells originating from the pallial ventricular zone (Emx1 positive), and a later developing population of GAGA-ergic cells. The glutamatergic neurons are present in association with the astroglia before the arrival of the first callosal axons. The population of GABA-ergic neurons, which originate from the medial and caudal domains of the ganglionic eminence, migrates to the midline just before the initial cingulate fibers begin to cross.[57] The glutamatergic neurons become organized within the midline glia in 3 superficial (dorsal), intermediate, and deep (ventral) layers (see **Fig. 1B**), a pattern further completed by later arriving GABA-ergic neurons. The cingulate and frontal callosal axons travel between the superficial and the intermediate layers, and the parietal callosal axons travel between the intermediate and the deep layers. The glutamatergic neuronal guideposts express Semaphorin3 (Sema3C) as an attracting guidance factor for the commissural axons[57]; they disappear by the time of birth (in mice), without any evidence of apoptosis, which suggests that they might migrate elsewhere. The GABA-ergic cell population seems to persist somewhat longer.[49,57] Primarily involved in the control of ciliogenesis, the transcription factor RFX3 (regulatory factor X3) is expressed in the glutamatergic neurons of the developing cortex and corpus callosum. It is has been shown to be required before the onset of callosal axon crossing for the patterning of the corticoseptal boundary; if RFX3 is inactivated, an inactivation of Gli3 and an increased expression of Nfg8 ensue and result in an abnormal distribution of the neuronal guideposts and a failure of the corpus callosum to develop properly.[58] The GABA-ergic population has been shown to express different combinations of guidance factors and cell adhesion molecules as well (described elsewhere in this article).[57]

These neuronal guideposts have been described in mice, not in humans. Interstitial callosal neurons have been observed in human brains, scarce at the beginning of the second trimester (ie, when the corpus callosum has become structurally complete) becoming more numerous afterward until the end of gestation. Their origin, and their function, are not clear, but the possibility that they derive from neuronal guidepost cells cannot be fully rejected.[59]

Commissural axonal guidance toward, across, and beyond the midline

Axons extend and find their way across the neural parenchyma by responding to guidance molecules. The tip of the axon forms a growth cone. The center of the growth cone is filled with microtubules that, by adding or removing tubulin segments, accompany the extension or retraction of the axon. The periphery of the growth cone is made of actin-rich lamellipodia with their filopodia. Filopodia are cytoplasmic extensions projecting in every direction, extending or retracting according to the molecular signals their transmembrane receptors get from the environment. By extending filopodia in response to an attractant signal and/ or by retracting them in response to a repellent signal, the growth cone may steer the progression of the axon across the tissue. Specific molecular signals are provided by specific cellular guideposts, and correspondingly specific axonal membrane receptors are needed for the axons to respond. Accordingly, axons may be guided toward local or distant ipsilateral targets, or toward a contralateral target, either heterotopically (decussations) or homotopically (commissures). Commissures are everywhere along the CNS, but because of the particularity of the telencephalic division with the presence of a tela choroidea and an associated telencephalic invagination, the development of the dorsal telencephalic commissure involves specific processes.

Once the callosal axons have been specified, the first step for them is to make the decision to extend to the midline rather than to ipsilateral targets; as discussed, this is regulated by *Neurogenin2* (*Ngn2*). The choice is made very early, just after the neuronal differentiation, meaning that the axon already proceeds medially well before the migration of the neuronal body into layers 2 and 3 is completed.[42] Also, neocortical commissural axons, which develop after, and follow the course of the pioneer cingulate commissural axons, travel toward the midline according to a low-lateral, high-medial gradient of *Sema3C* into the intermediate zone of the cingulate cortex where they fasciculate with the pioneer axons.[60,61]

When approaching, the axons are channeled toward the midline by the repulsive action of the indusium griseum glia dorsomedially and the glial wedge ventrolaterally, and attracted to the midline by the zipper astroglia and neuronal guideposts. Together, the indusium griseum glia and the glial wedge express repellent molecules: *Slit2* (receptor: *Robo*), *Wnt5a* (receptor: *Frizzled3*), and *Draxin* (receptor: *DCC*), which all prevent the callosal axons from extending locally in the adjacent midline cortex or septum pellucidum (where they would constitute the classical Probst's bundles); instead, they repel them toward the midline guideposts. Because the indusium griseum becomes ventrally dislocated in case of *Slit2* defect (as discussed), the callosal tract would be displaced ventrally also. In a similar way, the loss of *Draxin* would result in a lack of indusium griseum glia and be associated with the misrouting of the axons of all commissures. In the midline zipper astroglia and neuronal guideposts, the attractant *Semaphorin3* (*Sema3C*) is expressed by the calretinin-positive glutamatergic neurons, and its receptor *Neuropilin1* (Npn1) is expressed in the pioneer axons of the cingulate cortex; accordingly, the cingulate axons are conveyed across the midline. Npn1 is also expressed into the indusium griseum glia, however, and its role, therefore, may be more complex.[52] GABA-ergic neurons express *Sema3A* and *Npn2* receptors, *EphrinB1/B2*, and *EphB2/B3/A4* receptors, and adhesion molecules such as *Ncadh* and *Ncam1*.[57] Also, the usual Sema3A repulsive activity may be converted to attraction when Npn1 forms transmembrane interaction with *L1CAM*; it also depends on the cyclic

adenosine monophsophate/cyclic guanosine monophosphate ratio.[57] Similarly, the attractant *Netrin1* attracts the cingulate axons at the early stages of the commissuration, but not, later, the neocortical ones; it is not expressed in the midline glia, but rather in the adjacent cortex. Expressed in the callosal axons, its receptor DCC may actually be responding to the repulsive Draxin instead. This suggests that, rather than attracting the callosal axons, Netrin1 would act by decreasing their sensitivity to the contralateral Slit2 after crossing the midline, and therefore, allow them to proceed further toward their final cortical target.[60]

Indeed, the telencephalon with its guidance molecules is symmetric, which means that the postcrossing axons emerging from one hemisphere must reverse their responsiveness to the surrounding cues when entering the other hemisphere. The role of *Netrin1* in making the neocortical commissural axons insensitive to the repulsive influence of Slit2 immediately after the crossing is one example of such a process. Farther out in the hemisphere, it seems that the postcrossing neocortical callosal axons also lose their responsiveness to the cingulate cortex-derived Sema3C gradient, thanks to an upregulation of *Ephrin-B3*, which silences the response to Sema3C by binding to the Npn1 receptors and, therefore, reducing their availability.[60] In still another but quite similar way, it is interesting to point out that the commissural callosal axons crossing transversely the corticoseptal junction intersect with the parasagittal fibers of the septo-cingulate perforating pathway extending toward their ipsilateral cingulate targets, meaning that 2 tracts proceeding at the same time across the same location respond differently to the same local guiding cues.

Callosal axons cross sequentially, anterior cingulate pioneer axons first, then frontal and posterior temporoparietooccipital neocortical axons last. The latter proceed by fasciculation along the former, a process that involves the *L1CAM* molecule, a transmembrane protein more generally involved in the whole CNS in neuronal adhesion and neurite outgrowth and fasciculation. Cingulate and neocortical axons, however, remain segregated within the corpus callosum, with the former being located dorsally, and the latter, ventrally. Such a strict organization is likely needed for correct pathfinding toward the final contralateral cortical targets. It correlates the organization of the neuronal guideposts in 3 layers, as mentioned. It has also been shown to depend on *EphA3* signaling, a receptor that binds to the corresponding Ephrin ligand and is preferentially expressed in the lateral cortex.[62] How the axons in the final part of their course find their specific, usually homo-topic contralateral target is still not clear, with functional activity and the subsequent axonal pruning being likely involved.[63]

Finally, it must be mentioned that, although the corpus callosum attains its final shape at the beginning of the second trimester and is structur-ally complete by midgestation, the cortex by then is not completed and ready to be connected yet; the incoming callosal fibers have to remain con-nected to the neurons of the transient cortical sub-plate until much later in gestation, because the commissural/association final connections to the cortex itself in human fetuses does not occur until 32 weeks of gestation in the primary sensorimotor cortex, and still later, even postnatally, in the highly associative frontal regions.

THE HUMAN PATTERNS OF COMMISSURAL DYSGENESIS

For the clinical neuroradiologist, the data collected in mice contribute enormously to the understand-ing of the normal morphogenesis, but they cannot, in most cases, be related directly to the clinical malformative patterns. Even though it is estimated that approximately 40% of patients diagnosed with the malformation also present genetic abnor-malities or syndromic features,[64,65] few cases actually have been shown to be directly related to the metabolic pathways identified in mice. For instance, FGFR1 has been shown to play a major role in the development of the midline glia. FGFR defects are found in the syndromic craniosynosto-sis, but midline abnormalities are found mostly in the Apert syndrome (FGFR2 defect; **Fig. 2**); these changes also are relatively minor, far from the complete agenesis with Probst's bundle observed in the animal experiments.[66] Patients with a L1CAM defect present clinically with a CRASH syndrome (for Callosal agenesis, mental Retarda-tion, Adducted thumb, Spasticity, and Hydroceph-alus); however, the callosal agenesis in this syndrome is only a part of a diffuse, major defect of the white matter development also responsible for a huge and not necessarily hydrocephalic ven-triculomegaly (**Fig. 3**). Also, callosal dysgenesis may be observed in cases of fetal alcohol syndrome; ethanol has been shown to inhibit L1CAM-mediated neurite outgrowth.[67] Other than in those few examples, cases of syndromic commissural dysgenesis are probably the result of more complex alterations of still undeciphered genetic cascades. In addition, most of the cases of conventional commissural agenesis are not syndromic.

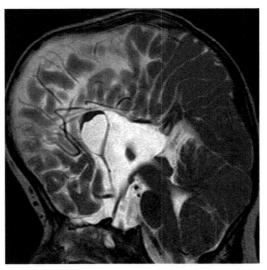

Fig. 2. Apert syndrome (FGFR2 defect). Incomplete commissural agenesis with absent (or diminutive) anterior commissure, absent hippocampal commis-sure, and hypogenetic anterior callosum with associ-ated septum pellucidum.

Conventional, sporadic cases of commissural agenesis as observed in clinical practice usually cannot be directly related to simple genetic de-fects either. Other than the missing callosum, the features of the classical complete agenesis of the corpus callosum often include in addition a missing anterior commissure, a missing hippocampal commissure, as well as a missing inferior cingulum and missing association

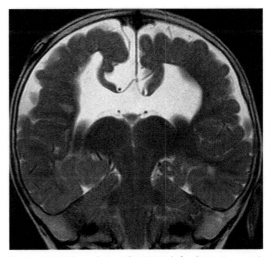

Fig. 3. CRASH syndrome (L1CAM defect). Huge ventri-culomegaly owing to the lack of most of the deep white matter; the septum pellucidum (including the fornix) and the corpus callosum are missing as well. The tela choroidea closes the ventricles dorsally.

bundles in the posterior part of the hemisphere (resulting in the classical colpocephalic appearance); the developmental defect is, therefore, more diffuse and less specific than would depend on the midline commissural apparatus only. Gobius et al[32] hypothesized that the retention of a deep interhemispheric cleft down to the tela choroidea would be the cause of the callosal commissuration failure, rather than its consequence, because it would reflect a failure of the midline glia to organize. The molecular defect would, therefore, be extrinsic (meningeal) rather than intrinsic (parenchymal)[32]; again, this does not explain why other, apparently unrelated bundles are missing as well. Whether the Probst's bundles are present or not is obviously significant, because it tells whether the callosal axons are simply rerouted or are missing altogether, which may mean an absence, or poor specification, of the callosal neurons, or a global defect of the commissuration processes. Also, cases diagnosed as complete callosal agenesis may demonstrate a missing anterior commissure, or a small one, or a normal one. These 3 patterns are likely to relate to 3 different mechanisms. Finally, the reasons for the lack of a well-defined cingulate gyrus in patients with a complete callosal agenesis (the so-called radiating midline sulcal pattern) are not clear either; it might just reflect the failure of the cingulate pioneer callosal axons to form or to project medially (Fig. 4).

The isolated absence of an anterior corpus callosum with normally present anterior and hippocampal commissures that is occasionally observed suggests that the cause could be a defect interhemispheric fusion along the corticoseptal boundary or an initial defect of the cingulate axons to cross. By contrast, the presence of a normally present posterior callosum in a patient with a semilobar holoprosencephaly may be explained by the normal development of the temporal lobes, with normal fimbriae and normal hippocampal commissuration that would allow a normal splenium to form by fasciculation. The anterior (frontal) callosum would not form because of the absence of an anterior interhemispheric fissure, septum pellucidum, and corticoseptal boundary, but the hippocampal commissure would be able to cross because a medullary velum is present transversely between the anterior undivided hemispheric cortex and the tela choroidea. Finally, the cases in which a small, hypoplastic anterior callosum is observed may be due to a defect of the septum pellucidum to develop properly.

Beside the cases of classical isolated—complete or partial—commissural agenesis, a second significant group of commissural ageneses are those associated with a dysplasia of the interhemispheric meninges, be it lipomatous or cystic. The simplest, and also the less common example of such a dysplasia, is the interhemispheric lipoma. It was observed that the more anterior the lipoma, the more complete the agenesis of the corpus callosum was. Presumably, an anterior lipoma located at the level of the septum and corticoseptal boundary would prevent the midline bridge from developing, preventing the subsequent commissuration; more posteriorly located lipoma are only splayed by the growing callosum, so displaying a curvilinear shape.[34] Importantly, this type of interhemispheric, juxtachoroidal lipoma should be differentiated from the cases of more anterior, often massive interhemispheric lipomas associated with a frontonasal dysplasia; frontonasal dysplasia as well as anterior basal cephaloceles are commonly associated with callosal abnormality, for unknown reasons, independent of the presence or absence of a midline lipoma.

The commissural agenesis with multicystic interhemispheric dysplasia is more complex than the interhemispheric lipoma. It is characterized by the presence of multiple congenital cysts located above the roof of the third ventricle. Histologically, these cysts may be choroidal, leptomeningeal, or dural. They do not typically communicate together, and therefore often present with different signals on MR imaging. They usually extend on one side of the falx and are typically associated with a unilateral hemispheric dysplasia, including a dysplastic cortex and an

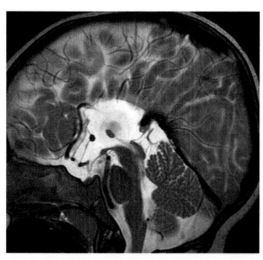

Fig. 4. Complete agenesis of the corpus callosum. Normal anterior commissure, but the hippocampal commissure is missing as well. The absence of a well-delineated cingulate gyrus is characteristic of the malformation.

often massive subcortical gray matter heterotopia (Fig. 5). On the normal side, the features are those of a classical agenesis with a Probst's bundle; on the dysplastic side, the Probst's bundle may be partial or absent, depending on the extent of the hemispheric malformation. In such cases, it is tempting to consider that the initial abnormal meningeal differentiation results in both the failure of the callosal fibers to cross, and the malformation of cortical development and heterotopia. This assumption that the meningeal disorder would be the cause of the commissural agenesis is supported by the uncommon cases of similar agenesis but without visible hemispheric abnormality. Alternatively, one may consider also that the dysplastic cortex is not receptive of the decussating fibers. The differentiation of the primitive meninge into its 3 pial, arachnoid, and dural layers occurs during the late embryonal period, starting ventrally to extend last at the interhemispheric fissure about week 8; this corresponds with the beginning of the commissuration process in humans.

The callosal agenesis with multiple interhemispheric meningeal dysplastic cysts must be distinguished from the uncommon pattern of a single, interhemispheric expansion of the prosencephalic tela choroidea (Fig. 6). Although forming an interhemispheric pouch, this expansion is continuous with the third and lateral ventricles. The falx may be normal or short. From these morphologic

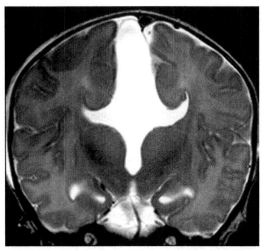

Fig. 6. Complete commissural agenesis with single interhemispheric expansion of the prosencephalic tela choroidea. Missing structures include the corpus callosum, the septum pellucidum (and Probst's bundles), and the fornices. The anterior and hippocampal commissures are lacking also (not shown). In contradistinction with the CRASH syndrome (see Fig. 3), the deep hemispheric white matter is otherwise normal.

features and from the fact that the corpus callosum, fornix, and septum pellucidum are all lacking, one may reasonably assume that the complete absence of the white matter along and

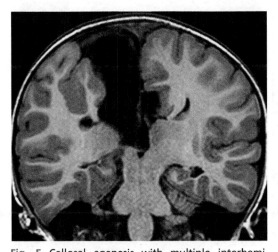

Fig. 5. Callosal agenesis with multiple interhemispheric cysts and subcortical gray matter heterotopia. Large right-sided, and smaller left-sided, interhemispheric meningeal cysts. Large right parietal subcortical heterotopia. Absent corpus callosum, with bilateral Probst's bundles, complete on the left, partial in the right presumably because of the gray matter heterotopia.

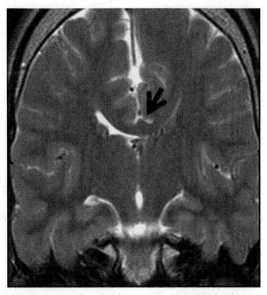

Fig. 7. Supracallosal ridge in a patient with Chiari 2 malformative complex. An abnormal white matter bundle is running on the dorsal aspect of the corpus callosum (black arrow), that has been identified as an aberrant crossing bundle of the dorsal cingulum.[67]

across the midline is the primary disorder, resulting in the choroidal expansion by a lack of containment.

The malformative complex of Chiari 2 usually associated with a myelomeningocele is not typically included in the syndromes associated with a callosal agenesis, and yet dysmorphic corpora callosa are common. The abnormalities may, together with the posterior lack of white matter, relate to a failure of the connectivity to develop properly owing to the congenital hydrocephalus. However, there are cases in which the corpus callosum is very short, suggesting a dysgenetic problem rather than a disruption of the development.[68] It has been demonstrated that in cases of early hydrocephalus, the radial glia may be compromised in the periventricular zones, resulting in the development of periventricular heterotopia[69] and, accordingly, periventricular heterotopia are not unusual in patients with Chiari 2; an early alteration of the periventricular progenitors/radial glia might affect the organization of the midline glial and neuronal guideposts as well.

Last, although some connections of the corpus callosum are known to be heterotopic, a large heterotopic callosal bundle (the so-called sigmoid bundle) is not classically described in normal anatomic studies. However, it has been observed in patients with partial callosal agenesis,[70] as if the posterior callosal axons that should normally have crossed along the hippocampal commissure were initially attracted toward a diminutive commissural plate at the frontal level and then attracted postcrossing by the local frontal guidance signals toward the local anterior cortex. A quite similar sigmoid bundle can be observed in patients with Chiari 2 malformation (and only rarely, in normal individuals) running over the dorsal surface of the corpus callosum, forming a dorsal ridge that seems to relate to an aberrant bundle of the dorsal cingulum (**Fig. 7**)[67]; the possibility that the initial pioneer axons would have taken an aberrant course can be considered. Finally, a last subtype of sigmoid bundle is observed in patients who present with a frontal lobar hemimegalencephaly; in this instance, however, the bundle is located at the level of the septum pellucidum, coursing from the abnormal frontal lobe to the posterior part of the contralateral hemisphere (or possibly, vice versa) and crossing the midline more ventrally than the normal course of the corpus callosum; the nature, origin, and crossing site(s) of this bundle are not identified (**Fig. 8**).

A   **B**

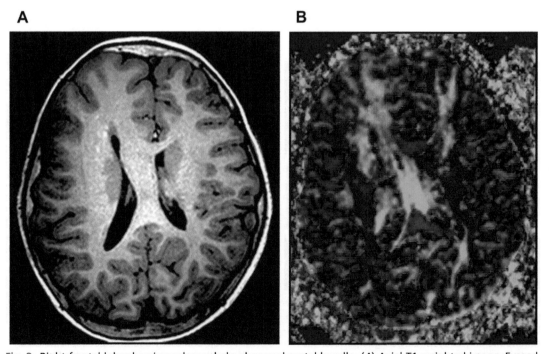

Fig. 8. Right frontal lobar hemimegalencephaly, abnormal septal bundle. (*A*) Axial T1 weighted image. Exceedingly thick septum pellucidum. (*B*) Fractional anisotropy map of the same plane: the septum pellucidum is occupied by a thick antero-posterior bundle of fibers directed toward the abnormal frontal lobe, and originating from the posterior left hemisphere.

REFERENCES

1. Vulliemoz S, Raineteau O, Jahaudon D. Reaching beyond the midline: why are human brains cross wired? Lancet Neurol 2005;4:87–99.
2. Abbie AA. The origin of the corpus callosum and the fate of the structures related to it. J Comp Neurol 1939;70:9–44.
3. Aboitiz F, Montiel J. One hundred million years of interhemispheric communication: the history of the corpus callosum. Braz J Med Biol Res 2003;36:409–20.
4. Gobius I, Suarez R, Morcom L, et al. Astroglial-mediated remodeling of the interhemispheric midline during telencephalic development is exclusive to eutherian mammals. Neural Dev 2017;12:9.
5. Castellani V. Building spinal and brain commissures: axon guidance at the midline. ISRN Cell Biol 2013;315387.
6. Rakic P, Yakovlev PI. Development of the corpus callosum and cavum septi in man. J Comp Neurol 1968;132:45–72.
7. Richards LJ. Axonal pathfinding mechanisms at the cortical midline and in the development of the corpus callosum. Braz J Med Biol Res 2002;35:1431–9.
8. Puelles L, Rubenstein JLR. Forebrain gene expression domains and the evolving prosomeric model. Trends Neurosci 2003;26:9.
9. Lamantia AS, Rakic P. Cytological and quantitative characteristics of four cerebral commissures in the Rhesus monkey. J Comp Neurol 1990;291:520–37.
10. Guénot M. Transfert interhémisphérique et agénésie du corps calleux. Capacités et limites de la commissure blanche antérieure. Neurochirurgie (Paris) 1998;44(Suppl 1):113–5.
11. Di Virgilio G, Clarke S, Pizzolato G, et al. Cortical regions contributing to the anterior commissure in man. Exp Brain Res 1999;124:1–7.
12. Wilson CL, Isokawa M, Babb TL, et al. Functional connections in the human temporal lobe. I. Analysis of limbic system pathways using neuronal response evoked by electrical stimulation. Exp Brain Res 1990;82:279–92.
13. Wilson CL, Isokawa M, Babb TL, et al. Functional connections in the human temporal lobe. II. Evidence for a loss of functional linkage between contralateral limbic structures. Exp Brain Res 1991;85:174–87.
14. Amaral DG, Insausti R, Cowan WM. The commissural connections of the monkey hippocampal formation. J Comp Neurol 1984;224:307–36.
15. Demeter S, Rosene DL, Van Hoesen GW. Interhemispheric pathways of the hippocampal formation, presubiculum and entorhinal and posterior parahippocampal cortices in the Rhesus monkey: the structure and organization of the hippocampal commissures. J Comp Neurol 1985;233:30–47.
16. Spencer SS, Williamson PD, Spencer DD, et al. Human hippocampal seizure spread studied by depth and subdural recording: the hippocampal commissure. Epilepsia 1987;28:479–89.
17. Gloor P, Salanova V, Olivier A, et al. The human dorsal hippocampal commissure. Brain 1993;116:1249–73.
18. Hofer S, Frahm J. Topography of the human corpus callosum revisited -Comprehensive fiber tractography using diffusion tensor magnetic resonance imaging. Neuroimage 2006;32:989–94.
19. Kier EL, Truwit CL. The lamina rostralis: modification of concepts concerning the anatomy, embryology, and MR appearance of the rostrum of the corpus callosum. AJNR Am J Neuroradiol 1997;18:715–22.
20. Velut S, Destrieux C, Kakou M. Anatomie morphologique du corps calleux. Neurochirurgie (Paris) 1998;44(Suppl 1):17–30.
21. Aboitiz F, Scheibel AB, Fisher RS, et al. Fiber composition of the corpus callosum. Brain Res 1992;598:143–53.
22. Widjaja E, Nilsson D, Blaser S, et al. White matter abnormalities in children with idiopathic developmental delay. Acta Radiol 2008;49:589–95.
23. Liss L, Mervis L. The ependymal lining of the cavum septi pellucidi: a histological and histochemical study. J Neuropathol Exp Neurol 1964;23:355–67.
24. Lancon JA, Haines DE, Lewis AI, et al. Endoscopic treatment of symptomatic septum pellucidum cysts: with some preliminary observations on the ultrastructure of the cyst wall: two technical reports. Neurosurgery 1999;45:1251–7.
25. Ronsin E, Grosskopf D, Perre J. Morphology and immunohistochemistry of a symptomatic septum pellucidum cavum Vergae cyst in man. Acta Neurochir 1997;139:366–72.
26. Shu T, Shen WB, Richards LJ. Development of the perforating pathway: an ipsilaterally projecting pathway between the medial septum/diagonal band of Broca and the cingulate cortex that intersects the corpus callosum. J Comp Neurol 2001;436:411–22.
27. Yakovlev PI, Locke S. Limbic nuclei of thalamus and connections of limbic cortex. III. Cortico-cortical connections of the anterior cingulate gyrus, the cingulum, and the subcallosal bundle in the monkey. Arch Neurol 1961;5:364–400.
28. Déjerine J. Anatomie des Centres Nerveux, Rueff, Paris, 1895-1901. Paris: Reprint Masson; 1980.
29. Le Douarin NM, Couly G, Creuzet SE. The neural crest is a powerful regulator of the pre-otic brain development. Dev Biol 2012;366:74–82.
30. Subramanian L, Remedios R, Shetty A, et al. Signals from the edges: the cortical hem and antihem in

telencephalic development. Semin Cell Dev Biol 2009;20:712–8.

31. Moldrich RX, Gobius I, Zhang J, et al. Molecular regulation of the developing commissural plate. J Comp Neurol 2010;518:3645–61.

32. Gobius I, Morcom L, Suarez R, et al. Astroglial-mediated remodeling of the interhemispheric midline is required for the formation of the corpus callosum. Cell Rep 2016;17:735–47.

33. Hankin MH, Schneider BF, Silver J. Death of the subcallosal glial sling is correlated with formation of the cavum septi pellucidi. J Comp Neurol 1988;272:191–202.

34. Raybaud C. The corpus callosum, the other great forebrain commissures, and the septum pellucidum: anatomy, development, and malformation. Neuroradiology 2010;52:447–77.

35. Creuzet SE. Neural crest contribution to the forebrain development. Semin Cell Dev Biol 2009;20:751–9.

36. Choe Y, Zarbalis KS, Pleasure SJ. Neural crest-derived mesenchymal cells require Wnt signaling for their development and drive invagination of the telencephalic midline. PLoS One 2014;9:2.

37. Choe Y, Siegenthaler JA, Pleasure SJ. A cascade of morphogenic signaling initiated by the meninges controls corpus callosum formation. Neuron 2012;73:698–712.

38. Hakanen J, Salminen M. Defects in neural guidepost structures and failure to remove leptomeningeal cells from the septal midline behind the interhemispheric fusion defects in Netrin1 deficient mice. Int J Dev Neurosci 2015;47:206–15.

39. Fame RM, MacDonald JL, Macklis JD. Development, specification and diversity of callosal projection neurons. Trends Neurosci 2011;34:41–50.

40. Alcamo EA, Chirivella L, Dautzenberg M, et al. Satb2 regulates callosal projection neuron identity in the developing cerebral cortex. Neuron 2008;57:364–77.

41. Fame RM, MacDonald JL, Dunwoodie SL, et al. Cited2 regulates neocortical layer II/III generation and somatosensory callosal projection neuron development and connectivity. J Neurosci 2016;36:6403–19.

42. Hand R, Polleux F. Neurogenin2 regulates the initial axon guidance of cortical pyramidal neurons projecting medially to the corpus callosum. Neural Dev 2011;6:30.

43. Bahi-Buisson N, Poirier K, Fourniol F, et al. The wide spectrum of tubulinopathies: what are the key features for the diagnosis ? Brain 2014;137:1676–700.

44. Mutch CA, Poduri A, Sahin M, et al. Disorders of microtubule function in neurons: imaging correlates. AJNR Am J Neuroradiol 2016;37:528–35.

45. Yagi H, Oka Y, Komada M, et al. Filamin A interacting protein plays a role in proper positioning of callosal projection neurons in the cortex. Neurosci Lett 2016;612:18–24.

46. Armentano M, Filosa A, Andolfi G, et al. COUP-TFI is required for the formation of commissural projections in the forebrain by regulating axonal growth. Development 2006;133:4151–62.

47. Shu T, Li Y, Keller A, et al. The glial sling is a migratory population of developing neurons. Development 2003;130:2929–37.

48. Richards LJ, Plachez C, Ren T. Mechanisms regulating the development of the corpus callosum and its agenesis in mouse and human. Clin Genet 2004;66:276–89.

49. Niquille M, Garel S, Mann F, et al. Transient neuronal populations are required to guide callosal axons: a role for Semaphorin 3C. PLoS Biol 2009;7:10.

50. Tole S, Gutin G, Bhatnagar L, et al. Development of midline cell types and commissural axon tracts require Fgfr1 in the cerebrum. Dev Biol 2006;289:141–51.

51. Shu T, Butz KG, Plachez C, et al. Abnormal development of forebrain midline glia and commissural projections in Nfia knock-out mice. J Neurosci 2003;23:203–12.

52. Piper M, Moldrich RX, Lindwall C, et al. Multiple non-cell-autonomous defects underline neocortical callosal dysgenesis in Nfib-deficient mice. Neural Dev 2009;4:43.

53. Sanchez-Camacho C, Ortega JA, Ocana I, et al. Appropriate Bmp7 levels are required for the differentiation of midline guidepost cells involved in corpus callosum formation. Dev Neurobiol 2011;71:337–50.

54. Amaniti EM, Hasenpusch-Theil K, Li Z, et al. Gli3 is required in Emx1+ progenitors for the development of the corpus callosum. Dev Biol 2013;376:113–24.

55. Magnani D, Hasenpusch-Theil K, Benadiba C, et al. Gli3 controls corpus callosum formation by positioning midline guideposts during telencephalic patterning. Cereb Cortex 2014;24:186–98.

56. Unni DK, Piper M, Moldrich RX, et al. Multipler Slits regulate the development of midline glial populations and the corpus callosum. Dev Biol 2012;365:36–49.

57. Niquille M, Minocha S, Hornung JP, et al. Two specific populations of GABAergic neurons originating from the medial and the caudal ganglionic eminences aid in proper navigation of callosal axons. Dev Neurobiol 2013;73:647–72.

58. Benadiba C, Magnani D, Niquille M, et al. The ciliogenic transcription factor RFX3 regulates early midline distribution of guidepost neurons required for corpus callosum development. PLoS Genet 2012;8:3.

59. Jovanov-Milosevic N, Petranjek Z, Petrovic D, et al. Morphology, molecular phenotypes and distribution

of neurons in developing human corpus callosum. Eur J Neurosci 2010;32:1423–32.

60. Mire E, Hocine M, Bazeliere E, et al. Developmental upregulation of Ephrin-B1 silences Sema3C/Neuropilin-1 signaling during post-crossing navigation of corpus callosum axons. Curr Biol 2018;28: 1768–82.

61. Fothergill T, Donahoo ALS, Douglass A, et al. Netrin-DCC signaling regulates corpus callosum formation through attraction of pioneering axons and by modulating Slit2-mediated repulsion. Cereb Cortex 2014;24:1138–51.

62. Nishikimi M, Oishi K, Tabata H, et al. Segregation and pathfinding of callosal axons through EphA3 signaling. J Neurosci 2011;31:16251–60.

63. Nishikimi M, Oishi K, Nakajima K. Axon guidance mechanisms for establishment of callosal connections. Neural Plast 2013;2013:149060.

64. Paul LK, Brown WS, Adolphs R, et al. Agenesis of corpus callosum: genetic, developmental and functional aspects of connectivity. Nat Rev Neurosci 2007;8:287–99.

65. Al-Hashim AH, Blaser S, Raybaud C, et al. Corpus callosum abnormalities: neuroradiological and clinical correlations. Dev Med Child Neurol 2016;58: 475–84.

66. Raybaud C, Di Rocco C. Brain malformation in syndromic craniosynostoses, a primary disorder of white matter: a review. Childs Nerv Syst 2007;23: 1379–88.

67. Bearer CF. L1 cell adhesion molecule signal cascades: targets for ethanol developmental neurotoxicity. Neurotoxicology 2001;22:625–33.

68. Miller E, Widjaja E, Blaser S, et al. The old and the new: supratentorial MR findings in Chiari II malformation. Childs Nerv Syst 2008;24:563–75.

69. Ferland RJ, Batiz LF, Neal J, et al. Disruption of neural progenitors along the ventricular and subventricular zones in periventricular heterotopia. Hum Mol Genet 2009;18:497–516.

70. Wahl M, Strominger Z, Jeremy RJ, et al. Variability of homotopic and heterotopic callosal connectivity in partial agenesis of the corpus callosum: a 3T diffusion tensor imaging and Q-Ball tractography study. AJNR Am J Neuroradiol 2009;30:282–9.

Moving?

Make sure your subscription moves with you!

To notify us of your new address, find your **Clinics Account Number** (located on your mailing label above your name), and contact customer service at:

Email: journalscustomerservice-usa@elsevier.com

800-654-2452 (subscribers in the U.S. & Canada)
314-447-8871 (subscribers outside of the U.S. & Canada)

Fax number: 314-447-8029

**Elsevier Health Sciences Division
Subscription Customer Service
3251 Riverport Lane
Maryland Heights, MO 63043**

ELSEVIER

Printed and bound by CPI Group (UK) Ltd, Croydon, CR0 4YY

03/10/2024

01040372-0010